Clinical Investigations
on the Move

Clinical Investigations
on the move

Authors: Andrew Walker, Lina Fazlanie and
Rory Mackinnon
Editorial Advisor: Ian Bickle
Series Editors: Rory Mackinnon, Sally Keat,
Thomas Locke and Andrew Walker

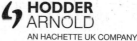

HODDER
ARNOLD
AN HACHETTE UK COMPANY

First published in Great Britain in 2012 by
Hodder Arnold, an imprint of Hodder Education, a division of Hachette UK
338 Euston Road, London NW1 3BH

http://www.hodderarnold.com

[Environmental statement to be inserted on all biblio pages and deleted by Production if using printers where statement is NOT true]
Hachette UK's policy is to use papers that are natural, renewable and recyclable products and made from wood grown in sustainable forests. The logging and manufacturing processes are expected to conform to the environmental regulations of the country of origin.

Whilst the advice and information in this book are believed to be true and accurate at the date of going to press, neither the author[s] nor the publisher can accept any legal responsibility or liability for any errors or omissions that may be made. In particular, (but without limiting the generality of the preceding disclaimer) every effort has been made to check drug dosages; however it is still possible that errors have been missed. Furthermore, dosage schedules are constantly being revised and new side-effects recognized. For these reasons the reader is strongly urged to consult the drug companies' printed instructions, and their websites, before administering any of the drugs recommended in this book.

British Library Cataloguing in Publication Data
A catalogue record for this book is available from the British Library

Library of Congress Cataloging-in-Publication Data
A catalog record for this book is available from the Library of Congress

ISBN-13   978-1-444-12154-4

1 2 3 4 5 6 7 8 9 10
Commissioning Editor: Joanna Koster
Project Editor: Stephen Clausard
Production Controller: Jonathan Williams
Cover Design: Amina Dudhia
Indexer: Laurence Errington

Cover image © GJLP/Science Photo Library
Typeset in 10/12 pt Adobe Garamond Pro Regular by Datapage
Printed and bound in India

What do you think about this book? Or any other Hodder Arnold title?
Please visit our website: www.hodderarnold.com

Contents

Preface

Have you ever found interpreting clinical investigations overwhelmingly complicated? Are you simply short of time and have exams looming? If so, this short revision guide will help you. Written by students and junior doctors, this book presents information in a wide range of formats including flow charts, summary tables and authentic images annotated with comments. During the course of writing this book, the students among us have now become qualified doctors ourselves.

Always remember to both request and review clinical investigations in the context of clinical findings. Medicine is both an art and a science, so be thoughtful and consider your findings prior to launching a further round of potentially expensive and futile investigations.

No matter what your learning style, we hope you will find this book appealing and easy to read. We think that this innovative style will help you, the reader, to connect with this often feared topic — helping you to learn and understand it (maybe even enjoy it!) while also helping to prepare you for exams and life as a junior doctor.

We of course welcome your feedback on how this book measures up and how you feel it could aid your study and work better. Every day is a new learning experience for us all.

AUTHORS:

Andrew Walker BMedSci MBChB — Specialist Trainee Year 1 doctor in Medicine, Chesterfield Royal Hospital, Chesterfield, Derbyshire, UK
Lina Fazlanie BMedSci MBChB — Foundation Year 1 doctor, Royal Hallamshire Hospital and University of Sheffield, UK
Rory Mackinnon BSc MBChB — Foundation Year 2 doctor, Northern General Hospital, Sheffield, UK

EDITORIAL ADVISOR:

Ian Bickle MB BCh BAO (Hons), FRCR — Consultant Radiologist, Department of Radiology, Raja Isteri Pengiran Anak Saleha Hospital, Bandar Seri Begawan, Brunei

EDITOR-IN-CHIEF:

Rory Mackinnon BSc MBChB – Foundation Year 2 doctor, Northern General Hospital, Sheffield, UK

SERIES EDITORS:

Sally Keat BMedSci MBChB – Foundation Year 1 doctor, Northern General Hospital, Sheffield, UK

Thomas Locke BSc MBChB – Foundation Year 1 doctor, Northern General Hospital, Sheffield, UK

Andrew Walker BMedSci MBChB – Specialist Trainee Year 1 doctor in Medicine, Chesterfield Royal Hospital, Chesterfield, Derbyshire, UK

Acknowledgements

The authors would like to thank the following people for their contribution towards the production of this book.

- Mr Kirtik A Patel MD, FRCS, Consultant Upper GI and Bariatric Surgeon, Northern General Hospital, Sheffield
- Dr Ian R Hall BSc(Hons), MD, MRCP, Consultant Cardiologist/Honorary Senior Clinical Lecturer, South Yorkshire Cardiothoracic Centre, Northern General Hospital, Sheffield
- Helen Heath, Clinical Nurse Educator, Coronary Care Unit, Northern General Hospital, Sheffield
- Sheffield Teaching Hospitals Foundation Trust

List of abbreviations

- AAA: abdominal aortic aneurysm
- ABCDE: Airway, Breathing, Circulation, Disability, Exposure
- ABG: arterial blood gas
- ACE: angiotensin-converting enzyme
- ACTH: adrenocorticotrophic hormone
- ADH: anti-diuretic hormone
- AFB: acid-fast bacilli
- AFP: α-fetoprotein
- alk phos, ALP: alkaline phosphatase
- ALL: acute lymphoblastic leukaemia
- ALP: alkaline phosphatase
- ALT: alanine aminotransferase
- AMA: anti-mitochondrial
- AML: acute myeloid leukaemia
- ANA: antinuclear antibody
- ANCA: anti-neutrophil cytoplasmic antibodies
- anti-GBM: anti-glomerular basement membrane
- AP: anteroposterior
- APTT: activated partial thromboplastin time
- ASOT: anti-streptolysin O titre
- AST: aspartate transaminase
- AVN: atrioventricular node
- BCP: basic calcium phosphate
- BJP: Bence–Jones protein
- CABG: coronary artery bypass grafting
- CEA: carcinoembryonic antigen
- CJD: Creutzfeldt–Jakob disease
- CK: creatine kinase
- CK-MB: creatine kinase-myocardial bound
- CLL: chronic lymphocytic leukaemia
- CLO: *Campylobacter*-like organism
- CML: chronic myeloid leukaemia
- CMV: Cytomegalovirus
- CNS: central nervous system
- COPD: chronic obstructive pulmonary disease
- CPPD: calcium pyrophosphate dihydrate
- CRH: corticotrophin-releasing hormone
- CSF: cerebrospinal fluid
- CSU: catheter sample of urine

- CSW: cerebral salt wasting
- CT: computed tomography
- CTPA: computed tomography pulmonary angiography
- CXR: chest radiograph
- DEXA: dual-energy X-ray absorption
- DI: diabetes insipidus
- DIC: disseminated intravascular coagulation
- DKA: diabetic ketoacidosis
- DM: diabetes mellitus
- DMARDs: disease-modifying anti-rheumatic drugs
- DVT: deep vein thrombosis
- EBV: Epstein–Barr virus
- EEG: electroencephalogram
- eGFR: estimated glomerular filtration rate
- ELISA: enzyme-linked immunosorbent assay
- EMG: electromyography
- ESR: erythrocyte sedimentation rate
- FBC: full blood count
- FEV_1: forced expiratory volume in 1 second
- FLAIR: fluid-attenuated inversion-recovery sequence
- FNA: fine needle aspirate
- FT_3: free T_3
- FT_4: free T_4
- FVC: forced vital capacity
- G6PD: glucose-6-phosphate dehydrogenase
- GGT/γ-GT: gamma-glutamyl transpeptidase
- GH: growth hormone
- GI: gastrointestinal
- GPAT: glycerol-3-phosphate acyltransferase
- Hb: haemoglobin
- HCT: haematocrit
- HDL: high-density lipoprotein
- HOCM: hypertrophic obstructive cardiomyopathy
- HONK: hyperosmolar non-ketotic coma
- HRCT: high-resolution computed tomography
- HSV: herpes simplex virus
- HU: Hounsfield unit
- IBC: iron binding capacity
- IDA: iron-deficiency anaemia
- IF: intrinsic factor
- Ig: immunoglobulin
- IGF: insulin-like growth factor
- IHD: ischaemic heart disease

- IM: intramuscular
- INR: international normalized ratio
- IV: intravenous
- IVU: intravenous urogram
- LAD: left anterior descending artery
- LCx: left circumflex artery
- LDH: lactate dehydrogenase
- LDL: low-density lipoprotein
- LFT: liver function test
- LKM-1: anti-liver/kidney microsomal-1
- MC&S: culture and sensitivity
- MCH: mean cell haemoglobin
- MCHC: mean cell haemoglobin concentration
- MCV: mean cell volume
- MDT: multidisciplinary team
- MI: myocardial infarction
- MRA: magnetic resonance angiography
- MRCP: magnetic resonance cholangiopancreatography
- MRI: magnetic resonance imaging
- MSU: midstream urine
- NSAID: non-steroidal anti-inflammatory drug
- NSTEMI: non-ST segment elevation myocardial infarction
- OGD: oesophagogastroduodenoscopy
- OGTT: oral glucose tolerance testing
- OSA: obstructive sleep apnoea
- PA: posteroanterior
- PAN: polyarteritis nodosa
- PCI: percutaneous coronary intervention
- PCOS: polycystic ovary syndrome
- PCR: polymerase chain reaction
- PJP: Pneumocystis *(carinii) jiroreci* pneumonia
- PE: pulmonary embolism
- PEA: pulseless electrical activity
- PEF: peak expiratory flow
- PKD: polycystic kidney disease
- Plt: platelets
- PMR: polymyalgia rheumatica
- PPI: proton pump inhibitors
- PSA: prostate-specific antigen
- PTH: parathyroid hormone
- PTHrP: parathyroid hormone-related peptide
- RA: rheumatoid arthritis
- RCA: right coronary artery

- RCDW: red cell distribution width
- RF: radiofrequency
- SIADH: syndrome of inappropriate antidiuretic hormone secretion
- SLE: systemic lupus erythematosus
- STEMI: ST-segment elevation myocardial infarction
- T_3: triiodothyronine
- T_4: thyroxine
- TB: tuberculosis
- TBG: thyroxine-binding globulin
- TIBC: total IBC
- TOE: transoesophageal echocardiography
- TPO: thyroid peroxidase
- TPPA: *Treponema pallidum* particle agglutination (assay)
- TRAb: thyrotrophin receptor antibodies
- TRHh: thyrotrophin-releasing hormone
- TSH: thyroid-stimulating hormone
- TTE: transthoracic echocardiography
- U+E: urea and electrolytes
- USS: ultrasound scan
- VDRL: venereal disease research laboratory
- VER: visually evoked responses
- VF: ventricular fibrillation
- VT: ventricular tachycardia
- VZV: varicella zoster virus
- WCC: white cell count
- WHO: World Health Organization
- α-FP: α-fetoprotein
- β-hCG: β-human chorionic gonadotrophin

An explanation of the text

The book is divided into three parts: common clinical investigations, clinical specialities and a self-assessment section. We have used bullet-points to keep the text concise and brief and supplemented this with a range of diagrams, pictures and MICRO-boxes (explained below).

MICRO-facts

These boxes expand on the text and contain clinically relevant facts and memorable summaries of the essential information.

MICRO-print

These boxes contain additional information to the text that may interest certain readers but is not essential for everybody to learn.

MICRO-case

These boxes contain clinical cases relevant to the text and include a number of summary bullet points to highlight the key learning objectives.

MICRO-reference

These boxes contain references to important clinical research and national guidance.

Normal range values are given for most tests in this book as a guideline for your knowledge. Please note that ranges differ between laboratories and therefore you should always use figures from your own institution to interpret results.

Part 1

Common clinical investigations

1 Haematology

1.1 FULL BLOOD COUNT

- The full blood count (FBC) is one of the most commonly requested investigations in hospital.
- Sample reference range are below – remember that parameters vary between institutions:

  haemoglobin (Hb)   11–14.7 g/dL (females); 13.1–16.6 g/dL (males)
  white cell count (WCC)   3.5–9.5 × 10^9/L
  platelets (Plt)   140–370 × 10^9/L
  haematocrit (HCT)   0.32–0.43 L/L (females); 0.38–0.48 L/L (males)
  mean cell volume (MCV)   80.0–98.1 fL (females); 81.8–96.3 fL (males)
  mean cell haemoglobin (MCH)   27.0–34.2 Pg
  mean cell haemoglobin concentration (MCHC)   33.5–35.5 g/dL
  neutrophils   1.7–6.5 × 10^9/L
  lymphocytes   1.0–3.0 × 10^9/L
  monocytes   0.25–1.0 × 10^9/L
  eosinophils   0.04–0.5 × 10^9/L
  basophils   0–0.1 × 10^9/L.

1.2 RED CELL DISORDERS: ANAEMIA AND POLYCYTHAEMIA

ANAEMIA

- Low Hb.
- Clinical signs include fatigue, pallor, breathlessness.
- Three key types, differentiated by MCV:
    - normocytic – red cells are normal size (MCV ↔);
    - microcytic – red cells are small (MCV ↓);
    - macrocytic – red cells are large (MCV ↑).
- Normocytic anaemias are related to:
    - acute blood loss
        - would become microcytic if there was chronic blood loss

- chronic diseases, e.g. rheumatoid arthritis
- haemolysis.

● Microcytic anaemias are related to:
  - iron-deficiency anaemia (IDA) – usually from chronic blood loss (commonly menorrhagia or gastrointestinal (GI) bleeding);
  - abnormal iron physiology, e.g. thalassaemia, sideroblastic anaemia.

● Macrocytic anaemias are due to:
  - impaired erythropoiesis, e.g. vitamin B_{12} or folate deficiency.
  - increased red cell production, as new erythrocytes are large (reticulocytes), e.g. haemolysis, cytotoxic chemotherapy.
  - alcohol abuse causing macrocytosis by both mechanisms:
    - direct toxic effect on erythrocytes, leading to increased production;
    - patients often have poor folate and B_{12} intake.

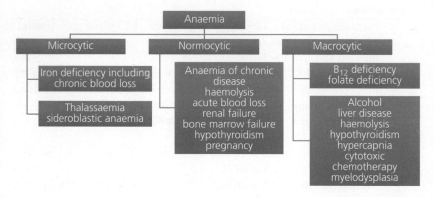

Fig. 1.1 Anaemias.

● Red cell distribution width (RCDW), although not routinely measured, gives an indication of the heterogeneity of the red cells within the blood. If elevated, it indicates that there may be two populations of red cells, i.e. a microcytosis and macrocytosis. In this case, the MCV may be normal.
● MCH and MCHC are useful to elucidate the cause of anaemia. A low value indicates hypochromic cells, associated with iron deficiency.

HAEMATOCRIT

● Erythrocytes make up approximately 35% of total blood in females, or 45% in males; the remainder is plasma and other cell types.
● The HCT is calculated by dividing the total volume of red cells by the total volume of blood.
● A high HCT indicates either a greater number of red cells in the blood (**polycythaemia**), or a decrease in the plasma volume (pseudopolycythaemia; also known as relative polycythaemia), e.g. due to dehydration.

Common clinical investigations

- A low HCT indicates anaemia, or may be due to fluid overload, e.g. excess administration of intravenous (IV) fluids.

Table 1.1 Haematocrit.

↑ HCT	↓ HCT
Polycythaemia	Anaemia
Chronic hypoxia, e.g. COPD, smoking, congenital heart disease	Fluid overload
Polycythaemia rubra vera	
Erythropoietin driven, e.g. ectopic production from tumours or erythropoietin abuse in athletes	
Pseudopolycythaemia	
Dehydration, e.g. burns	
Gaisböck's syndrome: chronic form of pseudopolycythaemia associated with obesity, hypertension and smoking	

IRON STUDIES

This group of tests is useful for assessing iron imbalances.
- Iron physiology (see Fig. 1.2):
    - Dietary **iron** is absorbed in the duodenum and jejunum and passes into blood.
    - Red cell breakdown in the liver and spleen also releases **iron** into the bloodstream.
    - It is transported in the blood bound to **transferrin**, which is produced by the liver.
    - It is deposited in the liver and other tissues and stored as **ferritin**.
    - It is transported to the bone marrow for erythropoiesis.

> ## MICRO-facts
> **Iron** is better absorbed with good levels of **vitamin C**, hence ascorbic acid is sometimes prescribed along with oral iron supplements.

- The following blood results show sample reference ranges for an iron profile: iron 8–33 μmol/L; % iron binding capacity (IBC) saturation 20–50%; total IBC (TIBC) 45–81 μmol/L; ferritin 30–400 ng/mL.

Common clinical investigations

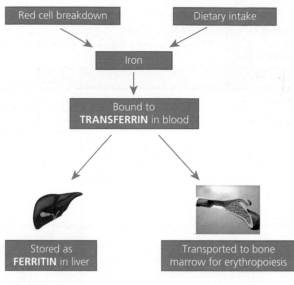

Fig. 1.2 Iron physiology.

> **MICRO-print**
> Note the % IBC saturation is calculated by dividing serum iron by TIBC and multiplying by 100.

- Causes of low iron:
  - chronic blood loss, e.g. from GI tract;
  - menorrhagia – very common;
  - malabsorption, e.g. Crohn's, or coeliac disease;
  - dietary – virtually impossible on Western die.
- Elevated iron levels may indicate haemochromatosis or haemolysis.
- Ferritin:
  - low in iron deficiency as stores are depleted;
  - high levels suggest haemochromatosis, or may be as a result of an acute illness – ferritin is an acute-phase reactant (see later under Erythrocyte sedimentation rate, and under C-reactive protein).
- TIBC:
  - an indirect measurement of transferrin;
  - may be increased in response to low iron levels.

Table 1.2 Examples of iron abnormalities.

CONDITION	IRON	FERRITIN	TIBC
Iron deficiency	↓	↓	↑
Sideroblastic anaemia	↑	↑	↔
Thalassaemia	↔	↔	↔
Haemochromatosis	↑	↑	↓

VITAMIN B_{12} AND FOLATE DEFICIENCIES

- Below are sample reference ranges for B_{12} and folate:
  - B_{12} 211–911 ng/L
  - folate deficient <3.4 µg/L; borderline 3.4–5.3 µg/L.
- B_{12} and folate deficiencies lead to macrocytic anaemias.
- B_{12} is absorbed in the terminal ileum.
- Intrinsic factor (IF) is required for B_{12} absorption and is produced by gastric parietal cells.

> ## MICRO-facts
> Iron, vitamin B_{12} and folate are known as the **haematinics**.

- Causes of B_{12} deficiency:
  - lack of IF
    - gastrectomy
    - autoimmune – pernicious anaemia;

> ## MICRO-facts
> The body's stores of B_{12} may last up to 3 years.

  - malabsorption
    - small bowel resection including terminal ileum
    - Crohn's, coeliac, tuberculosis (TB);
  - inadequate intake, e.g. eating disorders, alcoholism, dietary, e.g. veganism (rare).
- Specific tests for B_{12} deficiency:
  - immunological
    - anti-parietal cell antibody
    - anti-intrinsic factor antibody;
  - Schilling's test
    - Radiolabelled B_{12} is given orally, while ordinary B_{12} is given intramuscularly (IM).

Common clinical investigations

- Note that the normal IM B_{12} will not prevent the radioactive B_{12} from being absorbed from the gut, but should avoid the radioactive B_{12} from being stored, and hence promotes its excretion into the urine.
- Percentage of labelled B_{12} excreted is measured in a 24 hour urine sample. Percentage should be greater than 10%.
- If the percentage is low, the test is repeated with the additional administration of oral intrinsic factor.
- If the result normalizes, it is probably due to intrinsic factor deficiency, i.e. pernicious anaemia.
- If result is no better, the problem is due to malabsorption.
- **Folate** is absorbed throughout the small bowel.
- Causes of folate deficiency:
  - inadequate intake – including alcohol;
  - malabsorption – coeliac resection, Crohn's, tropical sprue, etc.;
  - drugs, especially folate antagonists, e.g. methotrexate, anti-epileptics, trimethoprim, sulfasalazine;
  - increased cell production – pregnancy, malignancy, inflammatory diseases, dialysis or chronic haemolytic anaemias.

MICRO-case

An 84-year-old woman presents to her GP with lethargy and worsening shortness of breath on exertion. On examination, she has pale conjunctivae, and is tachycardic. She appears to have lost weight. The GP orders a range of tests; the first to be reported is the FBC:

Haemoglobin   8.2 g/dL (normal 11–14.7 g/dL)
WCC 4.7×10^9/L (normal $3.5–9.5 \times 10^9$/L)
Platelets 280×10^9/L (normal $140–370 \times 10^9$/L)
Haematocrit   0.260 L/L (normal 0.32–0.43 L/L)
MCV   67.7 fL (normal 80.0–98.1 fL)
MCH   21.3 Pg (normal 27.0–34.2 Pg)
MCHM   31.5 g/dL (normal 33.5–35.5 g/dL)

Iron studies demonstrate a low serum iron, elevated TIBC and low ferritin. The GP orders a colonoscopy, which identifies caecal adenocarcinoma, and the patient is referred to the bowel cancer MDT meeting.

Learning points

- IDA is demonstrated by a microcytic, hypochromic picture on the FBC.
- The HCT will also be low.
- In elderly people, occult blood loss from the GI tract is the commonest cause of IDA.
- A history of steroid, aspirin or NSAID use should lead to suspicion of gastritis or peptic ulcer, requiring an OGD.
- Weight loss, lower abdominal pain or masses suggest colorectal malignancy, which can be investigated with colonoscopy.

HAEMOLYTIC ANAEMIAS

- Anaemia due to excessive red cell breakdown.
- Normocytic or macrocytic.
- Causes:
  - hereditary
    - G6PD (glucose-6-phosphate dehydrogenase) deficiency;
    - thalassaemia;
    - sickle cell anaemia;
    - spherocytosis;
    - pyruvate kinase deficiency.
  - acquired
    - autoimmune;
    - artificial heart valve;
    - malaria;
    - hypersplenism;
    - burns;
    - microangiopathic, e.g. sepsis with disseminated intravascular coagulation (DIC);
    - drugs;
      transfusion reaction;
    - maternal to fetal: ABO incompatibility, Rhesus D disease (now rare).
- Specific tests:
  - reticulocyte count ↑ due to increased red cell production;
  - bilirubin mildly ↑ due to red cell breakdown;
  - urinary urobilinogen ↑ due to red cell breakdown;
  - lactate dehydrogenase (LDH) ↑ due to red cell breakdown;
  - osmotic fragility test – for hereditary spherocytosis;
  - antiglobulin (Coombs') tests:
    - direct antiglobulin test is to detect autoimmune haemolytic anaemia;
    - indirect antiglobulin test is to detect haemolytic disease of the newborn (ABO).
  - blood film – red cell fragments, reticulocytes + +, abnormal cells, e.g. spherocytes.

1.3 WHITE CELL ABNORMALITIES

- Here are sample white cell reference ranges from the FBC:
  WCC $3.5–9.5 \times 10^9$/L
  neutrophils $1.7–6.5 \times 10^9$/L
  lymphocytes $1.0–3.0 \times 10^9$/L
  monocytes $0.25–1.0 \times 10^9$/L
  eosinophils $0.04–0.5 \times 10^9$/L
  basophils $0–0.1 \times 10^9$/L.

- Neutrophils, eosinophils and basophils are from the myeloid precursor cell, the **myeloblast**.
- Lymphocytes are from the lymphoid precursor cell, the **lymphoblast**.
- Monocytes are differentiated from **monoblasts**.

NEUTROPHILS

- Also known as polymorphs.
- Elevated number is a neutrophilia; insufficient number is a neutropenia.

Table 1.3 Neutrophil count disturbances.

↑ NEUTROPHILS	↓ NEUTROPHILS
Bacterial infection	Cytotoxic chemotherapy
Inflammation	Radiotherapy
Necrosis, e.g. post myocardial infarction	Sepsis
↑ Steroids: stress response (e.g. to surgery) or exogenous (e.g. prednisolone)	Bone marrow failure
Chronic myeloid leukaemia	Viral infection
	Hypersplenism including Felty's syndrome
	Drugs, e.g. carbimazole, clozapine

LYMPHOCYTES

Table 1.4 Lymphocyte count disturbances.

↑ LYMPHOCYTOSIS	↓ LYMPHOCYTOPENIA
Viral infection	Cytotoxic chemotherapy
Inflammation	Radiotherapy
Chronic lymphocytic leukaemia	Steroid treatment
Chronic infection, e.g. TB	Bone marrow failure
Atypical lymphocytes (Epstein–Barr virus infection)	HIV infection

OTHERS

- Eosinophils:
  - elevated in:
    - atopic/allergic conditions (e.g. asthma);
    - skin disorders (e.g. pemphigus);
    - parasitic infection (e.g. hookworm);
    - malignancy (e.g. Hodgkin's lymphoma);
    - hypereosinophilic syndrome (includes eosinophlia in association with hepatosplenomegaly and restrictive cardiomyopathy).
- Basophils:
  - raised in viral infections, inflammation, malignancies.
- Monocytes:
  - raised in viral infections, e.g. infectious mononucleosis, chronic illness, e.g. TB.

1.4 PLATELET DISORDERS

- Platelets are fragments of megakaryocytes and are responsible for clotting function.

Table 1.5 Platelet disturbances.

↑ THROMBOCYTOSIS	↓ THROMBOCYTOPENIA
'Reactive', i.e. in response to inflammation or infection	Autoimmune, e.g. idiopathic thrombocytopenia
Post splenectomy	Drugs, e.g. heparin (heparin-induced thrombocytopcnia)
Essential thrombocythaemia (myeloproliferative)	Bone marrow failure
Bleeding	↑ Usage, e.g. disseminated intravascular coagulation
Malignancy	Viral infections
Iron deficiency	

1.5 AN OVERVIEW OF HAEMATOLOGICAL DISORDERS

MYELOPROLIFERATIVE DISORDERS

- Disorders resulting in proliferation of mature cells from the myeloid line:
  - ↑ erythrocytes: polycythaemia rubra vera;

- ↑ white blood cells: chronic myeloid leukaemia;
- ↑ platelets: essential thrombocythaemia;
- ↑ bone marrow stromal cells: myelofibrosis.

ACUTE LEUKAEMIAS

- Two key types are acute myeloid leukaemia (AML) and acute lymphoblastic leukaemia (ALL).
- Acute leukaemias are characterized by malignant proliferation of *immature* precursor cells from the bone marrow.
- As such, **blast cells**: either **myeloblasts** or **lymphoblasts**, for AML and ALL respectively, will be present on the peripheral blood film and in bone marrow aspirate.
- Replacement of normal bone marrow cells with malignant cells leads to bone marrow failure and **pancytopenia** – a reduction in the levels of erythrocytes, white blood cells and platelets.

CHRONIC LEUKAEMIAS

- Two key types are chronic myeloid leukaemia (CML) and chronic lymphocytic leukaemia (CLL).
- Chronic leukaemias are characterized by malignant proliferation of *mature* blood cells.
- In CML: ↑ neutrophils, eosinophils, basophils.
  - Karyotyping for 'Philadelphia' chromosome may be performed – 95% of patients have this translocation of a section of DNA between chromosomes 9 and 22.
- In CLL: ↑ lymphocytes (usually B-cells).

LYMPHOMAS

- Abnormal malignant proliferation of lymphocytes.
- Distinct from lymphoid leukaemias because of lymph node involvement.
- Hodgkin's lymphoma:
  - ↑ lymphocytes, including Reed–Sternberg cells.
- Non-Hodgkin's lymphoma:
  - ↑ lymphocytes of another type – mostly B-cells.

MULTIPLE MYELOMA

- Malignant proliferation of plasma cells in bone marrow.
- These produce immunoglobulin, which may be found in blood and urine.
- Tests:
  - serum electrophoresis – looking for monoclonal bands;
  - 24-hour urine sample for Bence–Jones protein (BJP);

- bone marrow aspirate;
- ↑ ESR, ↑ Ca^{2+};
- radiological investigations may show lytic lesions, e.g. 'pepper-pot' skull.

1.6 CLOTTING SCREEN

- Here are sample reference values for a typical clotting screen:
  - prothrombin time (PT) 9.5–11.5 seconds
  - activated partial thromboplastin time (APTT) 25.5–37.5 seconds
  - fibrinogen 1.4–3.5 g/L.

PROTHROMBIN TIME (PT) AND THE INTERNATIONAL NORMALIZED RATIO (INR)

- **PT** is a measure of the function of the **extrinsic** pathway of coagulation.
  - PT is affected by levels and/or function of clotting factors I, II, V, VII and X.
  - Vitamin K is required for production of factors II, VII, IX and X, and thus deficiency leads to prolonged PT. Vitamin K is fat soluble.
  - Warfarin is a vitamin K antagonist, and thus prolongs PT.
- The international normalized ratio (INR) is a standardized measurement of a patient's PT against an internationally agreed, 'normal' standard.
  - It is calculated by dividing the patient's PT by the 'normal' PT, giving a ratio. Therefore a normal INR would be 1.
  - It is used to monitor warfarin therapy.

MICRO-facts

- The therapeutic range of **warfarin** is an **INR of 2–3** (i.e. 2–3 times the normal PT) for most indications, e.g. AF, DVT, PE.
- Metallic heart valves may need an **INR target of 3.5.**

- Causes of ↑ PT or INR:
  - warfarin (vitamin K antagonist);
  - liver disease (impaired clotting factor production);
  - cholestasis (lack of bile secretion and fat absorption, therefore ↓ vitamin K);
  - disseminated intravascular coagulation (DIC);
  - sepsis;
  - deficiency of factors I, II, V, VII or X;
  - heparin.

Common clinical investigations

ACTIVATED PARTIAL THROMBOPLASTIN TIME (APTT)

- The APTT is a measurement of the function of the **intrinsic** pathway of coagulation.
- It is affected by the function of all clotting factors except factor VII.
- An APTT ratio, similar to the INR, is used to monitor levels of unfractionated heparin. Note low molecular weight heparin has little effect on the APTT ratio.
- Causes of ↑ APTT:
  - heparin;
  - deficiencies of all clotting factors except VII:
    - e.g. haemophilia A + B;
    - specific factor deficiencies may be tested for if there is a prolonged APTT;
  - Von Willebrand disease;
  - lupus anticoagulant (will correct with Actin FS®);
  - liver disease;
  - DIC;
  - sepsis;
  - warfarin.

FIBRINOGEN

- An acute-phase reactant (see later under Erythrocyte sedimentation rate, and under C-reactive protein).
- Raised in any form of inflammation, infection.
- Low if:
  - excessive usage, i.e. clotting, for example in DIC;
  - decreased production, e.g. in liver disease.

MICRO-facts

Clotting screen and platelet levels are usually requested prior to surgery and interventional procedures such as biopsies.

1.7 OTHER HAEMATOLOGY TESTS

D-DIMER

- A product of clot degradation, therefore raised in cases of excessive clotting.
- Used for assessment of deep vein thrombosis (DVT) and pulmonary embolism (PE).
- Very non-specific – may be raised in a wide range of conditions, especially malignancy.

- A negative result makes PE and DVT unlikely, but should be interpreted in the clinical context.
- Causes of a raised D-dimer:
  - DVT or PE;
  - pregnancy;
  - infection;
  - inflammation;
  - malignancy;
  - peripheral vascular disease;
  - any convalescent hospital patient;
  - DIC.

> ## MICRO-facts
>
> D-dimer should be interpreted in the clinical context!

- May be artificially low if patient is on anticoagulant therapy.
- All results should be interpreted within the clinical context.
  - For example, in low probability of PE (as assessed according to British Thoracic Society guidelines) a negative D-dimer is sufficient to exclude PE.
  - In high probability of PE, D-dimer need not be performed – imaging (computed tomography pulmonary angiography (CTPA)) would be the first choice investigation.

> ## MICRO-reference
>
> British Thoracic Society guidelines for the management of suspected acute pulmonary embolism. **Thorax** 2003; 58: 470–83.

ERYTHROCYTE SEDIMENTATION RATE (ESR)

- An acute-phase reactant, elevated in inflammatory processes.
- May take several days for change in erythrocyte sedimentation rate (ESR) to reflect clinical condition.
  - Therefore good for management of chronic conditions, e.g. rheumatoid arthritis.
  - Less useful for assessment of response to treatment in acute infection, e.g. pneumonia.
- Elevated in:
  - infection;
  - inflammation:

- ↑↑ in vasculitis, particularly temporal arteritis;
- inflammatory arthritis, e.g. rheumatoid arthritis;
- connective tissue diseases, e.g. systemic lupus erythematosus (SLE), polymyalgia rheumatica (PMR);
- sarcoidosis
- malignancy – especially multiple myeloma.

C-REACTIVE PROTEIN (CRP)

- An acute-phase reactant, like ESR.
- Rises and falls according to clinical condition, much more quickly than ESR (within 48 hours).
  - Therefore, it is useful for assessment of response to treatment in acute infection.
  - It is less helpful for monitoring chronic diseases than ESR.
  - Elevated in: see earlier under Erythrocyte sedimentation rate.
  - Note that CRP is usually *not* elevated in SLE.

BLOOD FILM

- The blood film may be examined for evidence of many diseases.
- Thick and thin films may be used to identify the presence of malarial parasites.
- Routine blood films may show abnormal cells, e.g.:
  - reticulocytes – immature erythrocytes, present in IDA, post-chemotherapy, etc.;
  - hypochromic cells – IDA;
  - sickle cells – sickle cell anaemia;
  - spherocytes – hereditary spherocytosis, hyposplenism;
  - elliptocytes – hereditary elliptocytosis;
  - pencil cells – IDA;
  - poikilocytes – IDA, thalassaemia;
  - Heinz bodies – haemolysis in G6PD deficiency;
  - target cells – IDA, thalassaemia, liver disease;
  - blast cells – acute leukaemias (myeloblasts and lymphoblasts);
  - Auer rods – pathognomonic of AML.

BONE MARROW SAMPLING

- Used to diagnose haematological malignancies/myelodysplastic syndromes.
- May also elucidate cause of unexplained anaemias, e.g. show features of iron deficiency where other tests have been normal.
- Aspirate is useful to evaluate cellular content, while trephine is used for histological assessment.

Common clinical investigations

Clinical chemistry

2.1 UREA AND ELECTROLYTES AND RENAL FUNCTION

- Below are sample values for urea and electrolytes (U + E); remember these vary between institutions:

    sodium   134–143 mmol/L
    potassium 3.6–5.3 mmol/L
    urea   2.3–7.7 mmol/L
    creatinine 66–118 μmol/L.

> **MICRO-facts**
>
> U + E samples are not accurate if taken from an arm with an IV infusion running!

- One of the commonest tests ordered in hospital.
- Gives a basic measure of renal function.
- Elevated urea and creatinine demonstrate poor renal function.
- The absolute values are less important than the trend of change in a patient.
- Acutely raised urea with a normal or only mildly elevated creatinine implies gastrointestinal bleeding, as red blood cell breakdown increases serum urea, but not creatinine.

ESTIMATED GLOMERULAR FILTRATION RATE

- The estimated glomerular filtration rate (eGFR) gives a more accurate measure of renal function than urea and creatinine values alone.
- Not useful for acute changes in creatinine – see later under Creatinine clearance.
- Changes in a patient's eGFR value over time are more important than the absolute value compared with others.
- Based on:
    - serum creatinine;
    - age;

- sex;
- race.
- All results are standardized for a body surface area of 1.73 m^2.
- The normal value is ~100 mL/min/1.73 m^2.
- Reductions in this value are used as an indicator of overall renal function.

Table 2.1 Estimated glomerular filtration rate (eGFR) and chronic kidney disease (CKD).

eGFR (mL/min/1.73 m^2)	STAGE OF CKD	DESCRIPTION
>90	0–1	Normal kidneys unless other evidence present[a]
60–89	2	Mild impairment
45–59	3A	Moderate impairment
30–44	3B	
15–29	4	Severe impairment
<15	5	'End-stage' disease requiring dialysis or transplant (renal replacement therapy)

[a]If any of the following are present with an eGFR >90 mL/min/1.73 m^2 patient has Stage 1 CKD: proteinuria or haematuria; diagnosis of a genetic kidney disease, e.g. polycystic kidney disease; radiological evidence of structurally abnormal kidneys, e.g. reflux nephropathy.

MICRO-reference
http://www.renal.org/whatwedo/InformationResources/CKDeGUIDE.aspx (accessed 28/2/2011).

MICRO-print
Cautions with eGFR

- Not valid in pregnancy.
- Not valid for <18 years.
- Race should be taken into account – e.g. Afro-Caribbeans have a 20% greater eGFR than their Caucasian counterparts.

MICRO-facts
Assessment of eGFR or creatinine level is essential prior to IV contrast imaging investigations to prevent contrast-induced nephrotoxicity.

Common clinical investigations

CREATININE CLEARANCE

- This is useful for acute changes in renal function and for modifying doses of medications in acute renal impairment.
- A recent (i.e. within 24 hours) serum creatinine value is required.
- Use the following calculation:

$$(140 - \text{age}) \times \text{weight (kg)} / \text{serum creatinine (}\mu\text{mol/L)}$$
$$\times\ 1.04 \text{ female (or } 1.23 \text{ male)} = \text{CrCl mL/min}$$

2.2 SODIUM IMBALANCES

THIRST AXIS

- The hypothalamus regulates sodium and water balance.
- It detects changes in serum osmolality, which can be estimated with the following equation:

$$2(Na^+ + K^+) + \text{urea} + \text{glucose} = \text{serum osmolality}$$

MICRO-print
- Serum osmolality can also be measured directly in the laboratory.
- Differences between the estimated value and actual value may be due to the presence of poisons, e.g. salicylate, ethylene glycol.

- The normal range is 280–295 mosmol/kg H_2O.
- Antidiuretic hormone (ADH) is secreted by the posterior pituitary gland in response to high serum osmolality.
  - This increases reabsorption of water by the kidney, so lowering serum osmolality.
- Thirst is also activated at high serum osmolalities.
- There are four broad causes of an abnormal plasma sodium concentration.

Table 2.2 Sodium imbalances.

↓ PLASMA Na⁺ CONCENTRATION	↑ PLASMA Na⁺ CONCENTRATION
↑ Water, e.g. cardiac failure	↓ Water, e.g. dehydration
↓ Na⁺, e.g. thiazide diuretics	↑ Na⁺, e.g. excess 0.9% saline

HYPONATRAEMIA (Na⁺ <134 mmol/L)

In order to determine the most likely cause of a low serum sodium result, four other pieces of information are required:

Common clinical investigations

1) Patient's fluid status:
   - assessed clinically;
   - other information, e.g. haematocrit may be helpful (see Chapter 1, Haematology).
2) Serum osmolality (normal range 280–295 mosmol/kg H_2O).
3) Urine osmolality (high is >500 mosmol/kg H_2O).
4) Urinary sodium (high is >20 mmol/L).

Note that samples for serum and urine osmolality should be taken simultaneously.

- The causes of hyponatraemia may be classified first by the patient's fluid status, then differentiated with the other three results.

MICRO-facts

Key points for hyponatraemia

- Assessment of fluid status is crucial.
- Most causes of hyponatraemia lead to low serum osmolality.
- If serum osmolality is high, check glucose – osmotic effect is likely.
- If urine sodium is high, this suggests sodium loss is via the kidney.
- In hypovolaemia, if urine sodium is low, this suggests sodium loss from insensible losses.
- In fluid overload, values for all three tests will be low.

Table 2.3 Causes of hyponatraemia in the hypovolaemic patient.

CAUSE OF HYPONATRAEMIA	SERUM OSMOLALITY	URINE OSMOLALITY	URINE SODIUM
↑ Insensible losses, e.g. diarrhoea, fever	↓	↓	↓
Third-space losses, e.g. pancreatitis, burns	↓	↓	↓
Diuretics (+ + thiazides)	↔/↓	↑	↑
Osmotic effect, e.g. DKA, HONK	↑	↑	↑
Addison's disease (including iatrogenic)	↓	↑	↑
Salt-losing nephropathy	↓	↑	↑
Cerebral salt wasting	↓	↑	↑

DKA, diabetic ketoacidosis; HONK, hyperosmolar non-ketotic coma.

Table 2.4 Causes of hyponatraemia in the euvolaemic patient.

CAUSE OF HYPONATRAEMIA	SERUM OSMOLALITY	URINE OSMOLALITY	URINE SODIUM
Fluid therapy with insufficient Na$^+$, e.g. excess 5% dextrose	↓	↓	↓
SIADH	↓	↑	↑
Psychogenic polydipsia	↓	↓	↓
Hypothyroidism	↓	↑	↑
Hyperlipidaemia (pseudohyponatraemia)	↔/↑	↔	↔

SIADH, syndrome of inappropriate antidiuretic hormone secretion.

Table 2.5 Causes of hyponatraemia in the hypervolaemic patient.

CAUSE OF HYPONATRAEMIA	SERUM OSMOLALITY	URINE OSMOLALITY	URINE SODIUM
Cardiac failure	↓	↓	↓
Liver failure	↓	↓	↓
Nephrotic syndrome	↓	↓	↓
Renal failure	↔/↑	↔/↑	↑

SYNDROME OF INAPPROPRIATE ANTIDIURETIC HORMONE SECRETION (SIADH)

- The syndrome of inappropriate antidiuretic hormone secretion (SIADH) is a commonly diagnosed cause of hyponatraemia.
- Excessive ADH secretion causes low serum osmolality and high urine sodium and osmolality.
- Patients are euvolaemic.
- A diagnosis of exclusion – hypothyroidism and adrenal dysfunction must be excluded with thyroid-stimulating hormone (TSH) and 9 am cortisol (see later under Adrenal axis).
- Renal function must also be normal, and diuretics should not be involved.
- The causes are legion.
  - Tumours:
    - small cell lung cancer;
    - prostate;
    - thymus;
    - pancreas;
    - lymphomas;
    - brain.

- Pulmonary lesions:
  - small cell lung cancer;
  - pneumonia;
  - TB;
  - lung abscesses.
- Metabolic:
  - alcohol withdrawal;
  - porphyria.
- Central nervous system (CNS):
  - meningitis/encephalitis;
  - tumours;
  - head injury;
  - subdural haematoma;
  - cerebral abscess;
  - vasculitis, e.g. systemic lupus erythematosus (SLE).
- Drugs:
  - opiates;
  - antidepressants;
  - anticonvulsants;
  - cytotoxics;
  - proton pump inhibitors (PPIs) (rare).
- Although SIADH is common after head injury, cerebral salt wasting (CSW) is an important differential.
  - In SIADH patients are **euvolaemic**.
  - In CSW patients are **hypovolaemic**.
- Diagnostic criteria:
  - plasma osmolality <270 mosmol/kg H_2O;
  - urine osmolality >100 mosmol/kg H_2O;
  - patient is clinically euvolaemic;
  - elevated urinary sodium >40 mmol/l;
  - normal salt and water intake;
  - hypothyroidism, diuretic use and glucocorticoid deficiency excluded.

HYPERNATRAEMIA ($Na^+ >143$ mmol/L)

This is caused by either sodium excess or lack of water.

Table 2.6 Causes of hypernatraemia.

SODIUM EXCESS	LACK OF WATER
Excessive normal saline (0.9%)	Dehydration, e.g. burns, diarrhoea Diabetes insipidus ($\downarrow$ ADH)

ADH, antidiuretic hormone.

DIABETES INSIPIDUS

- Dehydration caused by lack of water retention by the kidney.
- Diabetes insipidus (DI) is either cranial or nephrogenic.
  - Cranial DI is due to lack of production of ADH:
    - caused by tumour, infection, trauma.
  - Nephrogenic is due to lack of effect of ADH on the kidney:
    - inherited or caused by renal disease, drugs (e.g. lithium), hypoka-laemia or hypercalcaemia.
- Diagnosis is by the water deprivation test.
  - The patient is deprived of water.
  - Serum and urine osmolality are measured at hourly intervals (paired).
  - Differentiates DI from psychogenic polydipsia.
  - Normal result (i.e. psychogenic):
    - serum osmolality remains normal;
    - urine osmolality increases to > 300 mosmol/kg H_2O;
    - ADH levels before and after water deprivation are then measured to confirm the finding.
  - DI result:
    - serum osmolality increases;
    - urine osmolality does not increase adequately;
    - administration of desmopressin (DDAVP®) differentiates cranial from nephrogenic DI:
      - ○ in cranial DI urine osmolality will increase;
      - ○ in nephrogenic DI urine osmolality will remain the same.

MICRO-case

An 85-year-old man who was previously fit and well is admitted with haemoptysis and weight loss. He has a history of cigarette smoking of 40 pack years. Routine bloods on admission showed the following:

sodium   117 mmol/L (normal 134–143 mmol/L)
potassium   4.7 mmol/L (normal 3.6–5.3 mmol/L)
urea   6.7 mmol/L (normal 2.3–7.7 mmol/L)
creatinine   116 μmol/L (normal 66–118 μmol/L).

The junior doctor on the ward assesses the patient's fluid status and concludes that the patient is euvolaemic. She takes a serum sample for osmolality just after the patient returns from passing a urine sample, which is sent for urine sodium and osmolality:

urine sodium   56 mmol/L (normal <20)
urine osmolality   546 mosmol/kg H_2O (normal <500)
serum osmolality   264 mosmol/kg H_2O (normal 280–295).

continued...

continued...

The patient also has a 9 am cortisol and thyroid function test, which both come back normal. He is not on any diuretic therapy.

The patient has a computed tomography-guided biopsy of a suspicious lesion identified on plain chest radiograph, which gives a tissue diagnosis of small cell lung cancer.

The patient is started on fluid restriction to 1 L in 24 hours. Within 2 weeks, his Na^+ is within the normal range.

Learning points

- SIADH is commonly associated with many lung pathologies, including small cell lung cancer. It is a common paraneoplastic syndrome.
- Serum and urine osmolalities should be paired, i.e. taken at as close to the same time as possible.
- To diagnose SIADH, renal, thyroid and adrenal function (as assessed by 9 am cortisol) must all be normal, and the patient should not be on diuretic therapy.
- Treatment is with fluid restriction, which may take a number of days/ weeks to correct the imbalance.
- Very severe, symptomatic hyponatraemia may be treated with demeclocycline, which causes iatrogenic nephrogenic diabetes insipidus, thus limiting the effect of ADH on the kidneys.

2.3 POTASSIUM IMBALANCES

HYPERKALAEMIA ($K^+ > 5.3$ mmol/L)

MICRO-facts

Potassium levels > 6.5 mmol/L or with **ECG changes** (see Chapter 6, Cardiovascular system) are a **medical emergency**, as ventricular arrhythmias are likely.

- Causes:
    - increased K^+ intake, e.g. inappropriate IV therapy;
    - cell breakdown, e.g. **haemolysed sample,** rhabdomyolysis, burns, tumour lysis syndrome (intracellular concentration of K^+ is much higher than extracellular);
    - renal failure;
    - drugs:
        - diuretics – especially spironolactone
        - angiotensin-converting enzyme (ACE) inhibitors;
    - Addison's disease;
    - acidosis, e.g. diabetic ketoacidosis.

HYPOKALAEMIA (K$^+$ < 3.5 mmol/L)

MICRO-facts

Potassium levels < **2.5 mmol/L or** < **3.0** with **ECG changes** (see Chapter 6, Cardiovascular system) are a medical emergency, as ventricular arrhythmias are likely.

- Causes:
    - diuretics, e.g. furosemide, bendroflumethiazide;
    - insufficient administration of K$^+$ in IV fluids;
    - diarrhoea/vomiting and hypovolaemia;
    - Cushing's syndrome or steroids;
    - Conn's syndrome;
    - alkalosis e.g. metabolic;
    - renal tubular acidosis;
    - salt-wasting renal disease;
    - drugs: insulin, salbutamol.

2.4 LIVER FUNCTION TESTS

- Below are sample reference values for liver function tests (LFTs):
    - total protein   63–79 g/L
    - albumin   35–48 g/L
    - globulin   18–36 g/L
    - total bilirubin   5–28 μmol/L
    - ▶

Table 2.7 Liver function tests.

TEST	MARKER OF SYNTHETIC FUNCTION	MARKER OF LIVER DAMAGE
Total protein	✓	
Albumin	✓	
Globulin	✓	
Total bilirubin	✓	
Alkaline phosphatase		✓
Aspartate transaminase (AST)		✓
Alanine aminotransferase (ALT)		✓
Gamma-glutamyl transpeptidase (GGT)		✓

Common clinical investigations

alkaline phosphatase   36–125 IU/L
aspartate transaminase (AST)   15–41 IU/L
alanine aminotransferase (ALT)   17–63 IU/L
gamma-glutamyl transpeptidase (GGT/γ-GT)   7–50 IU/L.

- Although commonly used, the term 'liver function test' is misleading; some of the tests included in an LFT profile measure synthetic products of the liver, but others are actually markers of liver damage (see Table 2.7).

PROTEIN

> ### MICRO-facts
>
> As the liver also synthesizes clotting factors, prothrombin time is a key marker of synthetic liver function (see Chapter 1, Haematology).

- The liver synthesizes **albumin** and some **globulins**.
- Other globulins are produced by immune cells (i.e. immunoglobulins).
- As such, **total protein**, **albumin** and **globulin** are markers of liver function.
- **Total protein** – **albumin** = **globulin** (approximate value).
- Any form of liver disease may lead to impaired protein synthesis.
- These are therefore non-specific indicators of hepatic dysfunction.
- **Albumin** levels are also decreased in:
  - sepsis and acute illness;
  - chronic illness, e.g. malignancy, autoimmune disease;
  - renal failure.
- Serum protein levels are affected by renal dysfunction:
  - decreased in nephrotic/nephritic syndromes due to loss in the urine;
  - decreased in fluid overload (dilutional);
  - increased in dehydration.
- **Total protein** and **globulin** may be elevated in malignancies that produce immunoglobulin, e.g. multiple myeloma.
  - a large gap between the total protein and the albumin levels would be evident.

HEPATITIC LFTs

- Hepatocellular damage releases liver enzymes into the bloodstream.
- The two most commonly measured markers of liver cell damage are the **transaminases:**
  - AST;
  - ALT.
- Causes of hepatitic LFTs:
  - infection, e.g. viral hepatitis;

- neoplasia – primary and secondary;
- degenerative, e.g. alcoholic liver disease – fatty liver, cirrhosis;
- metabolic, e.g. Wilson's disease, haemochromatosis;
- autoimmune hepatitis;
- vascular, e.g. congestive cardiac failure;
- iatrogenic – drugs, e.g. antifungals;
- toxins, e.g. excess paracetamol.

OBSTRUCTIVE LFTs

- Causes of obstructive LFTs may be divided by the location of the blockage.
  - In the lumen:
    - gall stone in bile duct.
  - In the wall:
    - cholangiocarcinoma;
      stricture of bile duct.
  - External:
      cholecystitis (infection of gall bladder with blockage);
    - ascending cholangitis – with raised white cell count (WCC), pain and pyrexia;
    - pancreatic malignancy (commonly head of pancreas);
    - enlarged lymph nodes near the porta hepatis, e.g. in malignancy/TB.
- Bilirubin:
  - If biliary outflow from the liver is obstructed, serum **bilirubin** will be elevated, leading to jaundice.
  - Assays to measure levels of **conjugated** and **unconjugated** bilirubin are available to differentiate obstructive (post-hepatic) from pre-hepatic causes of jaundice.
    - Bilirubin is conjugated in the liver to form bilirubin diglucuronide and therefore:
      - a high conjugated bilirubin would indicate post-hepatic obstruction;
      - a high unconjugated bilirubin level would indicate a pre-hepatic cause of jaundice, e.g. haemolysis.
- Alkaline phosphatase (alk phos, ALP):
  - Present in high levels in liver cells surrounding canaliculi, therefore serum levels are raised in obstruction as the cells are damaged by increased pressure.
  - Another isoform of **ALP** (bone alkaline phosphatase) is important in bone metabolism (see Chapter 3, Endocrinology).
  - Bone and liver isoforms may be measured separately if the cause of the abnormality is not clinically obvious.
- GGT:
  - Raised in obstruction.
  - Raised acutely particularly with alcohol abuse.

MIXED PICTURE

As with many things in medicine, the distinction between hepatitic and obstructive LFTs is not absolute.

- Severe obstruction causes back-pressure effects and hepatocellular damage, leading to raised hepatitic markers (transaminases).
  - Obstructive markers should be raised out of proportion to hepatitic markers in this case.
- Severe hepatocellular damage can lead to intrahepatic obstruction of bile.
  - Therefore bilirubin, ALP and GGT may be raised, e.g. in viral hepatitis or alcoholic liver disease.

> ### MICRO-facts
>
> When requesting imaging investigations it is essential to state the nature of LFT derangement (hepatitic, obstructive, mixed) to guide accurate investigation.

2.5 OTHER USEFUL TESTS

LIPIDS

- Total cholesterol:
  - This is a risk factor for ischaemic heart disease.
  - The test should be carried out when the patient is fasted.
  - The target level in those with ischaemic heart disease (IHD) is < 5.0 mmol/L.
  - For those with diabetes, cholesterol control is of paramount importance.
    - Target in diabetics is < 4.0 mmol/L.
  - Framingham IHD score should be used for overall assessment of cardiovascular risk.
  - Very high levels (> 7.5) with normal triglycerides implies familial hypercholesterolaemia.
  - Hypothyroidism may also cause elevated cholesterol.
  - See Chapter 6, Cardiovascular system, for further information.
- Total/high-density lipoprotein (HDL) cholesterol ratio:
  - A higher proportion of low-density lipoprotein (LDL) as opposed to HDL cholesterol confers a greater cardiovascular risk.
    - HDL levels are inversely correlated with IHD risk.
  - LDL cholesterol is not always measured directly, instead the HDL and total cholesterol are recorded, and a ratio produced.

- High-risk HDL levels:
  - <1.0 mmol/L males, <1.1 mmol/L females.
- Overall, total/HDL cholesterol ratio >5.0 confers greater than average risk of IHD.
- Triglycerides (normal <2.0 mmol/L):
  - May be raised with:
    - alcohol abuse;
    - diabetes;
    - familial lipid disorders.

> **MICRO-reference**
> National Institute of Clinical Excellence (NICE). Lipid modification. Cardio-vascular risk assessment and the modification of blood lipids for the primary and secondary prevention of cardiovascular disease. 2010; http://guidance.nice.org.uk/CG67/NICEGuidance/pdf/English (accessed 10/03/2011).

BICARBONATE AND CHLORIDE

- Below are sample reference values for bicarbonate (HCO_3^-) and chloride (Cl):
  bicarbonate   22–32 mmol/L;
  chloride   95 107 mmol/L.
- They are often measured as part of U + E.
- Serum (venous) bicarbonate allows assessment of pH:
  - low in acute acidosis as it buffers H^+ ions;
  - may be high in chronic acidosis, e.g. COPD, again as a buffer;
  - high in acute metabolic alkalosis;
  - less invasive than arterial blood gas sample for assessment of pH:
    - therefore useful in cases of DKA.
- Chloride, in combination with bicarbonate, sodium and potassium, may be used to calculate the anion gap (see Chapter 7, Respiratory medicine).

MAGNESIUM (0.70–1.00 mmol/L)

- Magnesium is important for cardiovascular function and for smooth muscle contraction.
  - High doses may be given in acute asthma or in polymorphic ventricular tachycardia (VT) also known as torsades de pointes.
- **Hypermagnesaemia** is rare.
  - Causes:
    - renal failure;
    - laxative/antacid abuse;
    - very rarely associated with treatment for the above conditions.

- **Hypomagnesaemia.**
  - Worsens hypocalcaemia, hypokalaemia, therefore if levels of these are low despite treatment, consider measuring Mg^{2+} levels.
  - Causes:
    - diarrhoea;
    - malabsorption, including re-feeding syndrome (see Chapter 3, Endocrinology);
    - short gut syndrome;
    - alcohol;
    - diuretics;
    - renal disease, e.g. acute tubular necrosis.

CREATINE KINASE (34–306 IU/L)

- Released during muscle breakdown, e.g.:
  - rhabdomyolysis;
  - myocarditis;
  - muscular dystrophy.
- Creatine kinase-myocardial bound (CK-MB) is more cardio-specific (see Chapter 6, Cardiovascular system) and may be used to indicate myocardial damage, e.g. infarction, myocarditis, etc.

LACTATE

- Elevated levels indicate anaerobic metabolism caused by hypoperfusion.
- May be measured on an arterial blood gas (ABG) sample for a rapid result.
  - Venous (serum) levels are usually more accurate.
- Used as a marker of prognosis in sepsis – levels >4 mmol/L indicate severe sepsis with shock and hypoperfusion.
- Lactic acidosis is a recognized complication of metformin therapy.
  - Patients with type II diabetes on metformin who are found to be acidotic on ABG should have a serum lactate measurement.
- Elevated levels are also associated with ischaemic causes of hypoperfusion, e.g. bowel ischaemia.

TUMOUR MARKERS

- Certain malignancies produce characteristic proteins, levels of which may be measured in the blood.
- Elevated levels of a tumour marker are not necessarily diagnostic of a particular malignancy, but may be used for screening, e.g. prostate-specific antigen (PSA).
- Tumour markers may also be used to monitor for recurrence of a malignancy after curative treatment, e.g. carcinoembryonic antigen (CEA) in bowel cancer.

Table 2.8 Common tumour markers and their indications.

TUMOUR MARKER	ASSOCIATED MALIGNANCY
Prostate-specific antigen (PSA)	Prostate
Carcinoembryonic antigen (CEA)	Colorectal and others including gastric, breast
CA-125	Ovarian and others including endometrial
CA-19-9	Pancreatic, colon
α-Fetoprotein	Hepatocellular, testicular
β-Human chorionic gonadotrophin	Testicular, trophoblastic, e.g. hydatidiform mole

MICRO-facts

Tumour markers are not diagnostic and should be requested and interpreted in the correct clinical context. Injudicious use is discouraged.

COMPLEMENT

- The cascade of complement proteins is part of the innate immune system.
- They form the membrane attack complex to destroy pathogens.
- Commonly measured proteins:
  - C3 is used up in infection, i.e. serum levels fall;
  - C4 remains relatively normal in infections.
- In autoimmune disease, e.g. lupus, **both** C3 and C4 are low.

IMMUNOGLOBULINS

- Immunoglobulins are antibodies produced by plasma cells (mature B cells).
- There are five types:
  - immunoglobulin (Ig) A:
    - found on mucosal surfaces;
    - deficiency is common and has little clinical significance;
    - involved in IgA nephropathy – deposition of immune complexes often after bacterial infection.
  - IgG:
    - commonest and smallest immunoglobulin;
    - elevated in acute infection, rising later than IgM, may also indicate previous exposure to a particular antigen;
    - deficiency leads to susceptibility to bacterial infection.

Common clinical investigations

- IgM:
  - largest immunoglobulin;
  - elevated early in acute infection and is gradually replaced by IgG.
- IgE:
  - involved in response to parasitic infection and allergy and is elevated in these conditions.
- IgD:
  - role is unclear.
- Serum electrophoresis and specific immunoglobulin levels may be used to investigate:
  - recurrent infection
    - may be due to immunoglobulin deficiency, e.g. IgG deficiency;
  - allergy
    - IgE levels;
  - haematological malignancy
    - multiple myeloma – abnormal plasma cells produce immunoglobulin, commonly IgG-like proteins (paraprotein), i.e. Bence–Jones protein;
    - Waldenstrom's macroglobulinaemia – IgM paraprotein found in blood;
    - both of these conditions may lead to hyperviscosity syndrome.
- Particular antibodies, e.g. hepatitis B surface antibody, may also be measured to detect immune response to specific infections (see Chapter 4, Microbiology).

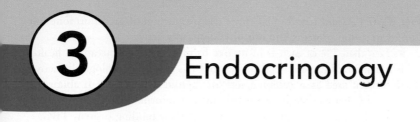

3 Endocrinology

3.1 THYROID AXIS

PHYSIOLOGY

> **MICRO-facts**
>
> **Reference ranges**
> TSH 0.35–4.5 mIU/L
> FT$_3$ 3.5–6.5 pmol/L
> FT$_4$ 10.0–19.8 pmol/L

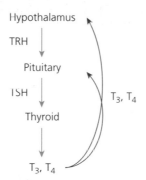

Fig. 3.1 Thyroid physiology. TRH, thyrotrophin-releasing hormone; TSH, thyroid-stimulating hormone; T$_4$, thyroxine; T$_3$, triiodothyronine.

- The hypothalamus secretes thyrotrophin-releasing hormone (TRH), which stimulates the pituitary to release thyroid-stimulating hormone (TSH).
- **TSH** causes the thyroid gland to release both thyroxine (T$_4$) and triiodothyronine (T$_3$).
- These both exert negative feedback on the pituitary and hypothalamus to maintain homeostasis.
- The thyroid hormones are bound to thyroxine-binding globulin (TBG) and albumin in the bloodstream.

- Free T_4 (FT_4), and free T_3 (FT_3) are the proportion of each hormone not bound to serum proteins and are physiologically active.
  - Less than 1% of each is in its free form in the bloodstream in health.
- T_4 is metabolized in peripheral tissues to T_3 as it is more biologically active.
- **TSH** is often used as a screening test for thyroid dysfunction. If abnormal, FT_3 and FT_4 may be done to provide further information.
- Levels of T_4 and T_3 are affected by those of their binding protein **TBG**.
  - TBG is raised in:
    - high levels of oestrogen, e.g. oral contraceptive pill, pregnancy;
    - hepatitis.
  - TBG is low in:
    - high levels of steroids – exogenous or Cushing's disease/syndrome;
    - nephrotic syndrome, i.e. protein loss in urine.

HYPERTHYROIDISM

- **Primary** causes:
  - Graves' disease (autoimmune);
  - toxic multinodular goitre;
  - toxic single thyroid nodule;
  - De Quervain's (subacute) thyroiditis.
    - Note this begins with hyperthyroidism, then hypothyroidism following once thyroid hormone stores are depleted.
  - post-partum thyroiditis;
  - drugs: amiodarone.

Table 3.1 Causes of hyperthyroidism.

CONDITION	TSH	FREE T_3/T_4
Graves' disease	↓	↑
Toxic multinodular goitre/toxic single nodule	↓	↑
De Quervain's thyroiditis (early phase)	↓	↑
Post-partum thyroiditis	↓	↑
Secondary hyperthyroidism (e.g. TSH-secreting pituitary tumour)	↔/↑	↑

TSH, thyroid-stimulating hormone; T_3/T_4 (triiodothyronine/thyroxine).

MICRO-print
Thyroid cancers almost never cause thyrotoxicosis; therefore, a palpable nodule in the presence of hyperthyroidism can be assumed to be a toxic, 'hot' nodule.

- **Secondary** causes:
  - TSH-secreting pituitary tumour.

HYPOTHYROIDISM

- Causes:
  - post treatment for thyrotoxicosis, e.g. thyroidectomy, radio-iodine treatment;
  - Hashimoto's thyroiditis;
  - De Quervain's thyroiditis (late phase);
  - drugs: including lithium, amiodarone;
  - malignancy;
  - congenital;
  - iodine deficiency (rare);
  - rarely, pituitary tumour (non-TSH secreting).

Table 3.2 Causes of hypothyroidism.

CONDITION	TSH	FREE T_3/T_4
Post thyrotoxicosis treatment	↑	↓
Hashimoto's disease	↑	↓
De Quervain's thyroiditis (late phase)	↑	↓
Secondary hypothyroidism (e.g. pituitary tumour)	↓	↓
Sick euthyroid syndrome	↓/↔	↓

TSH, thyroid-stimulating hormone; T_3/T_4 (triiodothyronine/thyroxine).

MICRO-facts

Sick euthyroid syndrome

- Thyroid function tests are often unreliable in acute illness: they may be artificially deranged.
- Often they may show low/normal TSH and low FT_3, FT_4 when the patient is actually **euthyroid.**
- If in doubt, repeat tests when the patient has recovered from their acute illness.

THYROID AUTOANTIBODIES

- Thyrotrophin receptor antibodies (TRAb)/thyroid-stimulating immunoglobulins (TSI):
  - stimulate the thyroid to release T_3 and T_4, leading to hyperthyroidism;
  - present in the majority with Graves' disease;
  - present in half of cases of subacute (De Quervain's) thyroiditis.

Common clinical investigations

- **Thyroglobulin antibody**, thyroid peroxidase (TPO) antibody:
    - present in Hashimoto's disease;
    - TPO may also be raised in Graves' disease.

RADIOLOGICAL INVESTIGATIONS IN THYROID DISEASE

- Ultrasound:
    - allows differentiation between hard and cystic nodules;
    - may be used for biopsy, usually fine needle aspirate (FNA), for tissue diagnosis to differentiate malignancy from, e.g. a toxic nodule.
- Nuclear medicine:
    - Technetium-99
        - shows location of areas of high activity within thyroid gland:
            - ○ diffuse if Graves' disease;
            - ○ localized to nodules in toxic multinodular goitre or toxic single nodule.
    - Radioactive iodine uptake
        - indicates levels of thyroid function:
            - ○ high in Graves' disease, toxic multinodular goitre;
            - ○ low in De Quervain's thyroiditis, Hashimoto's disease.
- Computed tomography (CT):
    - gold standard for assessment of retrosternal goitre and any compression of the trachea;
    - may be used for staging in disseminated thyroid malignancy.

3.2 DIABETES MELLITUS AND BLOOD SUGAR

DIAGNOSIS OF DIABETES MELLITUS AND INTERMEDIATE HYPERGLYCAEMIA

- Random serum glucose:
    - A random serum glucose level of >11.1 mmol/L is highly suggestive of diabetes mellitus (DM).
    - DM may be diagnosed with one random serum glucose value >11.1 mmol/L in those with symptoms of the disease.
    - Two random serum glucose values >11.1 mmol/L are required for diagnosis in asymptomatic patients.
    - In practice, those with an abnormal random serum glucose result often undergo further testing with fasting serum glucose and/or oral glucose tolerance testing (OGTT).
- Fasting serum glucose:
    - Fasting serum glucose >7.0 mmol/L is diagnostic of DM in symptomatic patients. Two values >7.0 mmol/L are required for diagnosis in asymptomatic individuals.

- Impaired fasting glucose (roughly equivalent to impaired glucose tolerance) is diagnosed with fasting glucose 6.1–6.9 mmol/L.
  - The World Health Organization (WHO) does not recognize this condition and requires the OGTT to be performed with this diagnosis to prove impaired glucose tolerance.
- OGTT:
  - This is the gold standard for diagnosis of DM and impaired glucose tolerance.
  - A total of 75 g of glucose is given orally in 300 mL of water after fasting for ~15 hours.
  - Serum glucose levels are measured at intervals after dose.
  - DM may be diagnosed in those with 2-hour post-dose serum glucose >11.1 mmol/L.
  - Impaired glucose tolerance (roughly equivalent to impaired fasting glucose) is diagnosed with 2-hour post-dose serum glucose 7.8–11.1 mmol/L.

Table 3.3 Diagnosis of hyperglycaemic conditions.

CONDITION	SYMPTOMS?	FASTING SERUM GLUCOSE	OGTT: 2-H GLUCOSE
Diabetes mellitus	Yes	One reading >7.0 mmol/L	One reading >11.1 mmol/L
	No	Two readings >7.0 mmol/L	Two readings >11.1 mmol/L
Impaired fasting glucose	n/a	6.1–6.9 mmol/L	n/a
Impaired glucose tolerance	n/a	6.1–6.9 mmol/L (with OGTT)	7.8–11.0 mmol/L

OGTT, oral glucose tolerance test.

MICRO-reference
World Health Organization. Definition and diagnosis of diabetes mellitus and intermediate hyperglycemia. 2006; http://www.who.int/diabetes/publications/en/ (accessed 10/03/2011).

MONITORING OF DIABETES MELLITUS

- Serum glucose measurements:
  - provide only a snapshot view of overall glycaemic control;
  - random serum glucose is useful in acute situations, e.g. to indicate diabetic ketoacidosis (DKA) or hyperosmolar non-ketotic coma (HONK).

Common clinical investigations

- BM glucose monitoring:
  - fingerprick to produce sample for analysis;
  - simple hand-held device;
  - useful for patient's daily monitoring and for a simple screening test for hyper/hypoglycaemia.
- Glycosylated (glycated) haemoglobin (HbA1c):
  - the percentage of haemoglobin A which is irreversibly bound to glucose;
  - this binding happens at any stage in the life of the red cell, so with their average life span being 120 days, one would expect changes in HbA1c over roughly a 60 day period;
  - gives a clear indication of long-term glycaemic control:
    - therefore is useful for assessing response to treatment;
  - target <7.4% to reduce complications.

HYPERGLYCAEMIA (RANDOM SERUM GLUCOSE >11.1 mmol/L)

- Emergency causes:
  - DKA
    - type I diabetics (very rare in type II);
    - serum glucose elevated, sometimes only modestly so;
    - metabolic acidosis on ABG or ↓serum HCO_3^-;
    - ketones in urine (dipstick test);
    - history over hours-days.
  - HONK
    - type II diabetics;
    - typically very high serum glucose >35;
    - very high serum osmolality >340 mosm/kg H_2O;
    - history over days-weeks.
- Other causes:
  - diabetes mellitus type I and II:
    - omitted/inadequate insulin/oral hypoglycaemic therapy;
    - acute illness e.g. infection.
  - gestational diabetes mellitus;
  - steroids:
    - exogenous, e.g. prednisolone;
    - endogenous – due to cortisol release in response to stress, e.g. surgery or from Cushing's disease/syndrome.

HYPOGLYCAEMIA (SERUM GLUCOSE <3.5 mmol/L)

> **MICRO-print**
> Whipple's triad required to diagnose hypoglycaemia:
> a. Low serum glucose.
> b. Symptoms of hypoglycaemia.
> c. Symptoms reverse when hypoglycaemia treated.
>   - It is possible to be asymptomatic with a low glucose.

- Diabetic causes:
    - excess insulin/oral hypoglycaemics (e.g. sulphonylureas);
    - insufficient calorie intake for treatment level;
    - intercurrent illness, e.g. sepsis.
- Non-diabetic causes:
    - sepsis;
    - liver failure;
    - intoxication;
    - drugs, e.g. quinine;
    - 'dumping syndrome' post bariatric surgery;
    - adrenal failure, e.g. Addison's disease;
    - factitious disorder (e.g. Munchausen's syndrome):
        - deliberate overdose with insulin/oral hypoglycaemics;
        - may be distinguished from insulinoma by measuring C-peptide.
    - C-peptide is attached to endogenous insulin stored in the pancreas;
    - if serum insulin levels are high, but C-peptide levels are normal, this suggests exogenous insulin administration, i.e. factitious disorder;
    - insulinoma (rare)
        - C-peptide and insulin levels would be raised.

3.3 CALCIUM METABOLISM

PHYSIOLOGY

- Calcium (Ca^{2+}) and phosphate (PO_4^{3-}) are mainly stored in bone.
- Calcium is largely bound to albumin in blood.
    - **Corrected calcium** adjusts to give a more accurate calcium value in cases of hypoalbuminaemia.
    - In severely low albumin, **ionized (free) calcium** may be measured.
- Vitamin D:
    - increases intestinal absorption of both calcium and phosphate;
    - in vitamin D excess, serum levels of Ca^{2+} and PO_4^{3-} are elevated;
    - in vitamin D deficiency, serum levels of Ca^{2+} and PO_4^{3-} are low.

- Parathyroid hormone (PTH):
  - causes resorption of calcium from bone into bloodstream;
  - causes increased excretion of phosphate by the kidney.
- Alkaline phosphatase (alk phos/ALP):
  - a marker of bone turnover.
- Note that bone ALP is a different isomer to that found in the liver. In cases where the source of an elevated ALP is unclear, each isomer may be measured specifically.

HYPERCALCAEMIA (>2.6 mmol/L)

- If serum calcium elevated, measure PTH.

Table 3.4 Differential diagnosis of hypercalcaemia.

↑ PTH	↓ PTH
Primary hyperparathyroidism	Malignancy, e.g. myeloma
Tertiary hyperparathyroidism	Excess vitamin D/calcium intake
Familial benign hypocalciuric hypercalcaemia rare	Paget's disease of bone
	Sarcoidosis
	Hyperthyroidism

PTH, parathyroid hormone.

- **Secondary hyperparathyroidism** is a physiological adaptation to chronic low calcium, e.g. in renal failure.
- It leads to hypertrophy of the parathyroid glands and therefore:
  - ↑ PTH;
  - ↓ or ↔ serum calcium.
- **Tertiary hyperparathyroidism** results from chronic secondary hyperparathyroidism, e.g. in renal failure.
- It leads to hyperplasia of the parathyroid glands and therefore:
  - ↑ PTH;
  - ↑ serum Ca^{2+}.

HYPOCALCAEMIA (<2.2 mmol/L)

- If low serum calcium, check albumin, magnesium, phosphate, renal function and PTH.
  - In **hypoalbuminaemia**, serum calcium will be falsely low, therefore use corrected or ionized calcium (see earlier under Physiology).
  - In **hypomagnesaemia** (chronic), PTH secretion and action is impaired, therefore serum calcium will be low.
  - **Nephrotic/nephritic** syndromes may lead to hypoalbuminaemia.
  - **Chronic renal failure** may lead to secondary hyperparathyroidism and renal osteodystrophy. Phosphate will be elevated in this case.

Table 3.5 Differential diagnosis of hypocalcaemia.

↑ PTH	↓ PTH
Chronic renal failure	Iatrogenic hypoparathyroidism (thyroid/parathyroid surgery/radio-iodine)
Vitamin D deficiency (osteomalacia) (dietary, ↓ sun exposure, malabsorption, etc.)	Primary hypoparathyroidism
Acute pancreatitis	Hypomagnesaemia
Pseudohypoparathyroidism (PTH resistance)	Pregnancy (↓albumin)

PTH, parathyroid hormone.

PHOSPHATE IMBALANCES

- Hyperphosphataemia ($PO_4^- > 1.5$ mmol/L):
  - ↑ gastrointestinal (GI) intake, e.g. phosphate enema;
  - cell breakdown:
    - tumour lysis syndrome;
    - rhabdomyolysis;
    - haemolysis;
  - renal disease, e.g. chronic kidney disease (CKD);
  - hypoparathyroidism.
- Hypophosphataemia ($PO_4^- < 0.8$ mmol/L):
  - renal loss:
    - diuretics;
    - hyperparathyroidism;
  - inadequate GI intake:
    - starvation;
    - malabsorption;

Common clinical investigations

- alcoholism;
- antacids;
- redistribution:
  - ↑ insulin, e.g. re-feeding syndrome;
  - acute respiratory alkalosis.

MICRO-print
Re-feeding syndrome

- Common in hospitals.
- Occurs after a prolonged period of starvation, e.g. patients nil-by-mouth due to stroke, surgery etc.
- Excess insulin is released when re-feeding begins.
- This leads to:
  - hypophosphataemia;
  - hypomagnesaemia;
  - hypokalaemia.
- Treatment is phosphate replacement in the first instance – other levels will not normalize until hypophosphataemia is corrected.

BONE DISEASES

Table 3.6 Summary of blood results from some common bone diseases.

BONE DISEASE	CALCIUM	PHOSPHATE	ALKALINE PHOSPHATASE
Osteoporosis	↔	↔	↔
Osteomalacia	↓/↔	↓	↑
Paget's disease of bone	↔	↓	↑↑
Bone metastases	↑	↑	↑
Chronic kidney disease	↓	↑	↑

3.4 ADRENAL AXIS

PHYSIOLOGY

- The hypothalamus secretes corticotrophin-releasing hormone (CRH).
- The pituitary secretes adrenocorticotrophic hormone (ACTH).
- The adrenal glands secrete **cortisol,** which acts on both the pituitary and the hypothalamus via negative feedback.
- Aldosterone, important for sodium and water balance, is secreted by the adrenal cortex and is regulated via the renin–angiotensin system.

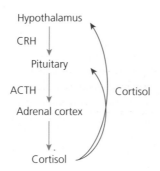

Fig. 3.2 Adrenal physiology. ACTH, adrenocorticotrophic hormone; CRH, corticotrophin-releasing hormone.

ELEVATED CORTISOL AND CUSHING'S SYNDROME

- Glucocorticoid excess has wide-ranging systemic symptoms and signs, collectively termed **Cushing's syndrome**.
- Exogenous cortisol from long-term glucocorticoid therapy (e.g. prednisolone) is a common cause of Cushing's syndrome.
- Endogenous causes:
  - pituitary microadenoma secreting ACTH – **Cushing's disease**;
  - primary adrenal adenoma secreting cortisol – rare;
  - ectopic ACTH secretion (paraneoplastic), e.g. small cell lung cancer.

Screening tests for Cushing's disease

- Serum cortisol (sample normal range: am, 198–720 nmol/L; pm, 85–459 nmol/L):
  - gives a snapshot of adrenocortical activity;
  - is usually measured at 9 am as levels should be near-peak at this point;
  - day curves can be measured to find maximal levels in patients with known Cushing's disease;
  - an elevated level should lead to further testing (see under section Diagnostic tests for Cushing's disease).
- Salivary cortisol:
  - a recent development and now the preferred screening test in many centres;
  - most sensitive screening test;
  - less invasive than blood sampling, which may cause a stress response and therefore an artificially high cortisol level;
  - usually measured at 11 pm, around which time one would expect the nadir in cortisol levels to occur;
  - an elevated level should lead to further testing (see under section Diagnostic tests for Cushing's disease).

Diagnostic tests for Cushing's disease
- 24-hour urinary-free cortisol:
  - an easy, straightforward test;
  - urine is collected for 24 hours and total cortisol is measured;
  - elevated level is usually considered diagnostic of Cushing's disease, although a dexamethasone suppression test may be done also;
  - more sensitive than a dexamethasone suppression test.
- Dexamethasone suppression test:
  - exogenous glucocorticoid in the form of dexamethasone acts on the adrenal axis via negative feedback;
  - this should lead to low measured cortisol levels in health;
  - there are two commonly used formats:
    - overnight dexamethasone suppression test – dexamethasone is given at 11 pm, serum cortisol is measured the following morning at 9 am;
    - low-dose dexamethasone suppression test – dexamethasone is given at 6 hourly intervals and serum and urine levels are measured at 0 and 48 hours;
  - elevated cortisol levels are diagnostic of Cushing's disease;
  - this test has the highest specificity of any of the investigations listed.

ADRENAL FAILURE AND ADDISON'S DISEASE

- Adrenal failure gives a characteristic picture on U + E testing:
  - $\downarrow Na^+$;
  - $\uparrow K^+$ (due to lack of aldosterone);
  - $\downarrow$ glucose.
- Primary adrenal failure:
  - addison's disease – autoimmune destruction of adrenal gland;
  - adrenal damage, e.g. metastases, TB.
- Secondary adrenal failure:
  - pituitary failure and therefore low ACTH levels lead to hypoadrenalism;
  - potassium may be normal as aldosterone is not affected.
- Iatrogenic:
  - Exogenous glucocorticoid therapy, e.g. prednisolone supresses endogenous production of ACTH.
  - If such therapy is stopped abruptly, there is no endogenous ACTH to stimulate adrenal cortisol production.
  - This therefore leads to a similar picture to that found in secondary adrenal failure.
  - Tapering down steroids with an appropriate reducing regime is therefore key to avoiding this complication.

- Short Synacthen® test:
  - Synacthen is synthetic ACTH.
  - Serum cortisol is measured, usually at 9 am.
  - 250 µg of Synacthen is given IV.
  - Serum cortisol is measured 30 minutes after the dose.
  - If serum cortisol is <550 nmol/L, this is consistent with an inadequate response by the adrenals to ACTH, i.e. primary hypoadrenalism.
  - The short Synacthen test will be normal in secondary hypoadrenalism.
- ACTH levels:
  - These will be low in secondary hypoadrenalism.
- Imaging, e.g. computed tomography (CT), may be used to characterize an adrenal mass, while magnetic resonance imaging (MRI) would be the best imaging modality to investigate a pituitary lesion.

3.5 OTHER ENDOCRINE INVESTIGATIONS

URINARY CATECHOLAMINES AND METANEPHRINES

- These are present in **phaeochromocytoma**.
- This is a tumour of the adrenal medulla in one or both glands releasing catecholamines, e.g. adrenaline.
- 24-hour urine sample for catecholamines and metanephrines; the breakdown product of catecholamines gives diagnosis.
- Ultrasound or CT scan may be used to characterize the tumour.

CONN'S SYNDROME INVESTIGATION

- This is an aldosterone-secreting adrenal tumour.
- Hypertension and hypokalaemia are common findings.
- Plasma **renin** levels may be measured, which are **low** in Conn's syndrome.

PROLACTIN

- Prolactin levels may be elevated with a pituitary microadenoma secreting the hormone.
- MRI may be used to characterize such a lesion.
- Prolactin may also be raised in polycystic ovary syndrome (PCOS).

ACROMEGALY

- Levels of growth hormone (GH) or insulin-like growth factor (IGF)-1 will be elevated.
- GH is antagonistic to insulin, and therefore type 2 diabetes mellitus is associated with this condition.
- The most accurate test is the 75-g oral glucose tolerance test. This should lower serum GH levels below 2 ng/mL in normal adults.

4 Microbiology

4.1 INVESTIGATION OF COMMON INFECTIONS

INTRODUCTION

- Basic investigations can give an indication of infection:
  - temperature – pyrexia, especially spiking or swinging, implies infection;
  - other vital signs may be affected, e.g. tachycardia, hypotension;
  - white cell count may be elevated in many conditions (see Chapter 1, Haematology) but within the appropriate clinical context it implies infection:
    - neutrophilia – likely bacterial infection;
    - lymphocytosis – likely viral infection.
- As a general rule, if you suspect infection in an area of the body, you should aim to obtain a sample from that area for analysis, e.g.:
  - suspected pneumonia, obtain sputum;
  - suspected urinary tract infection, obtain urine;
  - suspected meningitis, obtain cerebrospinal fluid, etc.
- Deep-seated infection, e.g. liver abscess, which does not respond to appropriate antibiotic therapy should be investigated with imaging and then be drained or excised as appropriate.
- All samples should be collected in a sterile fashion so as to avoid contamination with commensals from either the patient or the collector. The following are all helpful in minimizing contamination:
  - hand washing;
  - alcohol wipes/sterilizing solutions, e.g. chlorhexidine;
  - sterile equipment.

BACTERIAL INFECTION

- Microscopy:
  This is performed on most specimens, e.g. sputum, cerebral spinal fluid, to assess for the presence of bacteria and to differentiate them via their morphology and with specialist stains.

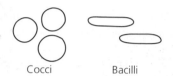

Cocci   Bacilli

Fig. 4.1 Bacterial morphology.

- **Cocci** – spherical bacteria, e.g.:
  - staphylococci, e.g. *Staphylococcus aureus*, found in clumps;
  - streptococci, e.g. *Streptococcus pneumoniae*, found in pairs (diplococci) or chains;
  - neisseria, e.g. *Neisseria meningitidis*, found in pairs.
- **Bacilli** – rod-shaped bacteria, e.g.:
  - *Escherichia coli*;
    Helicobacter pylori.
- Gram staining
  - Gram-positive – blue/purple, e.g. *Staphylococcus* species;
  - Gram-negative – red, e.g. *Escherichia coli*, *Klebsiella* species.
- Given the source of the specimen and simple microscopic findings, empirical antibiotic therapy can be chosen based on the likely pathogens identified.
- Culture and sensitivities:
  - Culture in ideal growing conditions may be performed in order to attempt to grow bacteria present in small quantities in the sample.
  - Culture media are treated with different antibiotics likely to affect a particular bacterium.
    - Areas of the media where the bacteria do not grow therefore have antibiotics sensitive to the pathogen.

VIRAL INFECTION

Investigation for viral infections may be done in two ways.
1) identify the virus itself, e.g. via amplification of viral DNA/RNA;
2) identify a host response to the virus, e.g. investigation for the presence of antibodies to a particular virus.

There are many techniques for the investigation of viruses, some of which are listed below. Some of these tests may also be used to investigate bacterial infections.

- Polymerase chain reaction (PCR):
  - This amplifies viral DNA/RNA.
  - This may be used to detect the presence of a particular virus, e.g. HIV.
- Enzyme-linked immunosorbent assay (ELISA):
  - This detects the presence of an antigen or antibody.

- An antigen or antibody is linked to an enzyme and added to the sample.
- If the corresponding antigen or antibody is present then an antigen–antibody–enzyme complex will be formed.
- This can be demonstrated by adding enzyme substrate and detecting the subsequent enzyme activity (for example, the colour of the solution may change).
- Serology testing:
  - This is an investigation for specific antibodies to a particular viral antigen.
  - Immunoglobulin (Ig)M antibodies are elevated in acute infection.
  - IgG antibodies are elevated in acute infection, but rise later than IgM. They may also indicate previous exposure.

4.2 INVESTIGATION OF SPECIFIC INFECTIONS

Below are some common tests for specific infections. The list is by no means exhaustive.

- Legionella urinary antigen:
  - To detect infection with *Legionella pneumophilia*, a cause of atypical pneumonia.
  - Urine is analysed for evidence of the bacterium.
- Mycoplasma GPAT (glycerol-3-phosphate acyltransferase):
  - To investigate for *Mycoplasma pneumoniae*, another cause of atypical pneumonia.
- Antistreptolysin O titre (ASOT):
  - Elevated in recent infection with streptococci.
- Thick and thin blood films:
  - To investigate for the presence of malarial parasites in blood.
- Auramine-phenol stain:
  - To look for acid-fast bacilli (AFB) on microscopy such as *Mycobacterium tuberculosis* (TB).
  - Ziehl–Neelsen staining is an older investigation for the same purpose.
  - If AFBs are identified, they can then be sent for culture and sensitivity, which may take up to 6 weeks.
- VDRL (venereal disease research laboratory) test:
  - For investigation of suspected syphilis (*Treponema pallidum*).
  - Other tests include specific serum IgM and *Treponema pallidum* particle agglutination assay (TPPA).
- Monospot test:
  - A rapid test for suspected Epstein–Barr virus (EBV).
  - EBV IgM is now more commonly used as the first-line investigation for recent infection as it is more sensitive and specific than the monospot test.

MICRO-case

A 35-year-old woman is seen in the GP surgery with dysuria and frequency which started the preceding evening. She is diagnosed with cystitis and is prescribed trimethoprim. Before she takes the antibiotic, she gives the doctor a urine sample that is dipstick-positive for nitrites and leucocytes.

Microscopy shows a Gram-negative bacillus, in keeping with an infection caused by *E. coli*, which is usually sensitive to trimethoprim.

After 48 hours the patient still has the same symptoms despite antibiotic therapy and contacts her GP. Her doctor checks the culture and sensitivity report for the urine and finds the following report:

E. coli viable count:
trimethoprim R (resistant);
amoxicillin R;
nitrofurantoin S (sensitive);
co-amoxiclav S.

The GP prescribes co-amoxiclav and the patient goes on to make a full recovery.

Learning points

- Empirical antibiotic therapy can be chosen based on the most likely pathogen suspected – *E. coli* is the commonest cause of urinary tract infection.
- Microscopy findings may help selection of the best empirical therapy.
- Culture and sensitivity allow the use of targeted antibiotic therapy.
- This allows antibiotic choices to be rationalized to avoid the prolonged use of broad-spectrum agents which increase resistance.

5 Radiology

5.1 PLAIN RADIOGRAPHS

BASIC INFORMATION

- Indications:
    - Signs and symptoms are potentially related to the respiratory, cardiovascular, musculoskeletal, genitourinary or gastrointestinal (GI) systems.
    - Follow-up of known disease, e.g. renal calculi.
    - Compliance with government regulations (e.g. immigration chest radiographs).
    - Note that there are some symptoms that are NOT indications for plain radiographs, e.g.:
        - acute GI blood loss – endoscopy would be the best investigation;
        - a palpable mass – computed tomography (CT) or ultrasound scan (USS) would be employed depending on site;
        - constipation – this should be a clinical diagnosis;
        - biliary disease – USS would be the first-line test.
- Contraindications:
    - There are no absolute contraindications.
    - Pregnancy in the first or second month is a relative contraindication; however, a shield may be placed on the abdomen in necessary cases.
- Preparations:
    - Ideally, all jewellery worn at the site of radiographic capture should be removed.
    - The patient is dressed in a hospital gown.
    - For a chest radiograph, the radiographer positions the patient next to the X-ray machine and asks them to take a deep breath and hold it for a few seconds while the radiograph is taken.
- Adverse effects:
    - There are no significant adverse effects. One plain chest radiograph is equivalent to 3 days of background radiation in the UK.
    - With these levels of radiation, carcinogenic and genetic effects cannot be ruled out, but remain merely theoretical risks.

PROJECTION

There are many projections of radiographs available; note that these descriptions may be combined, e.g. a mobile supine film.

MICRO-facts

The majority of chest radiographs are PA. If the radiograph fails to state the projection, then it is presumed a PA projection by default.

- Posteroanterior (PA):
  - Front of patient's chest against the film with the X-ray beam directed through the back.
- Anteroposterior (AP):
  - X-ray beams enter through the front of the chest and exit through the back.
  - The heart lies closer to the anterior chest wall, appearing artificially larger in this view due to magnification. Cardiac size and mediastinal contour is therefore difficult to assess.
  - Used when patients are too ill or immobile to facilitate a PA film; however, they offer a more limited interpretation.
- Lateral:
  - Often used in musculoskeletal radiographs to assess for fractures in two planes of view (termed orthogonal views).
  - Allows localization of an abnormality found on a chest PA film, but rarely used now with the common availability of CT scans.
- Expiratory (with regards to chest radiographs):
  - The patient is exhaling while the radiograph is taken.
  - Allows a pneumothorax to become more evident, but now rarely necessary.
- Inspiratory (with regards to chest radiographs):
  - The majority of radiographs require good inspiration to expand the lungs.

MICRO-print

Apical, oblique and lateral decubitus projections of the chest radiograph also exist; however, these are virtually obsolete due to the availability of CT scans.

MICRO-facts

On a PA projection of a chest film, the medial border of the scapula is more lateral as the patient 'hugs' the photographic plate, displacing the scapulae laterally. This method can be used to differentiate between PA and AP films.

Common clinical investigations

- Supine:
  - Taken while the patient is lying on their back.
  - Reserved for extremely ill patients who cannot sit up/stand.
  - Heart size is difficult to assess on this projection.
- Semi-erect:
  - The patient is upright, but not in an ideal position (e.g. sitting down).
- Erect:
  - The patient is upright.
  - Allows detection of gas in suspected bowel perforation on a plain chest radiograph as gas rises and accumulates below the diaphragm.
- Mobile:
  - Also known as 'portable'.
  - Taken using a mobile unit, often producing poorer quality films with longer exposure times.

MICRO-facts

Only request mobile radiographs when patients cannot be moved safely or appropriately to the radiology department.

DENSITIES OF PLAIN RADIOGRAPHS

- A plain radiograph image is produced by the projection of X-ray beams onto a plate/digital detector after passing through the patient.
- The body tissues therefore absorb the X-ray beams, with the residual radiation hitting the radiographic plate to produce an image.
- There are five main densities seen on plain radiographs: gas, fat, soft tissues, bone/calcified structures and artefacts.

Table 5.1 Densities of plain radiographs.

STRUCTURE ON RADIOGRAPH	SHADE
Artefacts	Intense white
Bone/calcified structures	White
Soft tissue	Grey
Fat	Darker grey
Gas	Black

BASIC ANATOMY FOR INTERPRETING CHEST RADIOGRAPHS

To interpret chest radiographs it is important to recognize the basic anatomical landmarks.

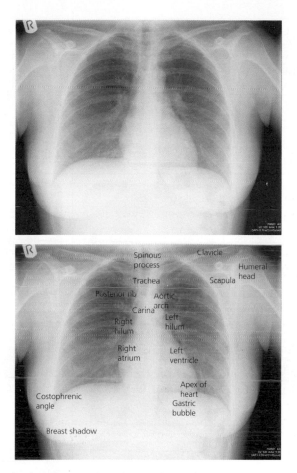

Fig. 5.1 Basic landmarks on a plain chest radiograph.

- The lungs:
  - Lobes of the lung
    - the right lung is divided into three lobes by the horizontal and oblique fissures;
    - the left lung is divided into two lobes by the oblique fissure.
  - Structures which should be identifiable in normal, translucent lungs are:
    - blood vessels;
    - interlobular fissures;
    - walls of larger bronchioles seen end-on (look circular).
  - The hilar shadows represent the pulmonary arteries and veins.
    - lung hila should be visible on either side;
    - the right hilum is slightly lower and larger than the left (maximum 1–2.5 cm lower).

Lobe	Frontal view	Lateral view
Right upper lobe	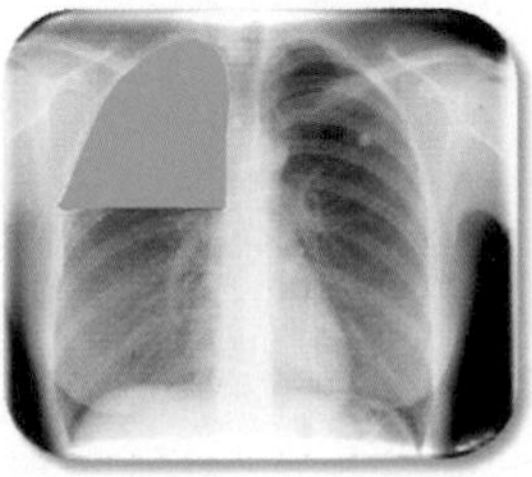	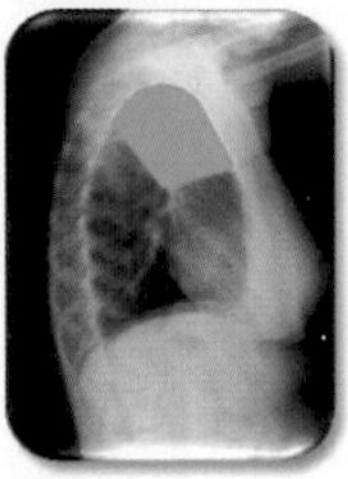
Right middle lobe	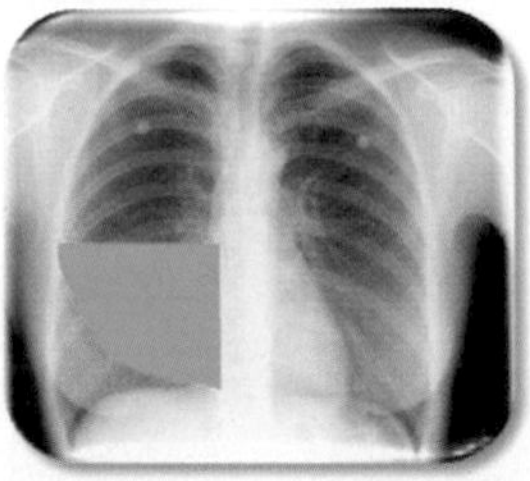	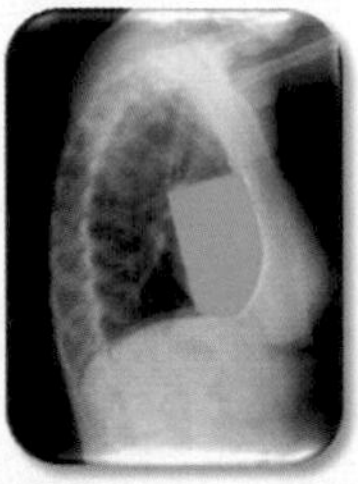
Right lower lobe	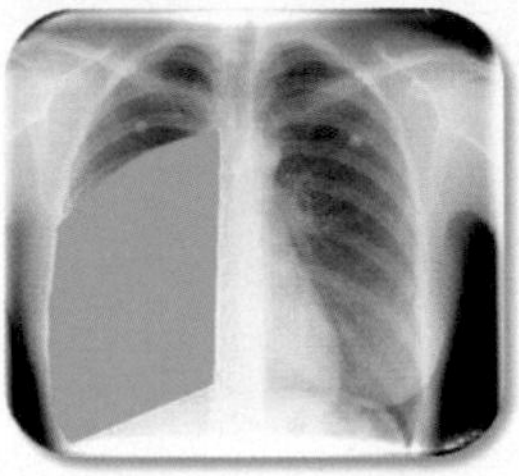	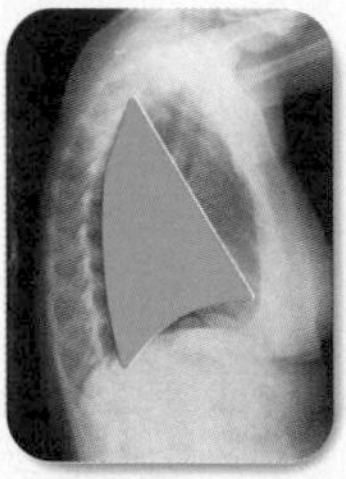
Left upper lobe and lingula	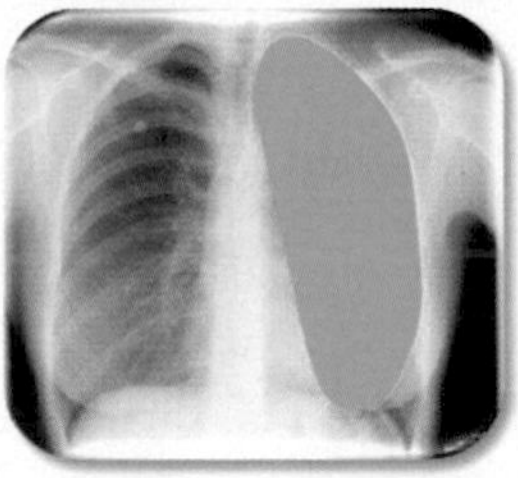	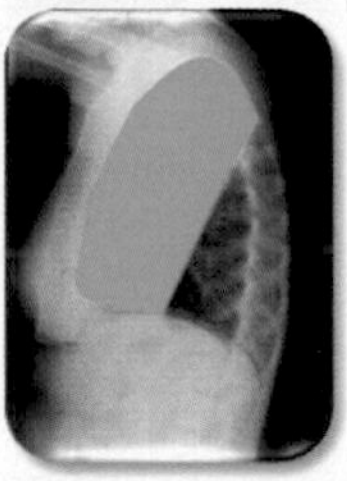
Left lower lobe	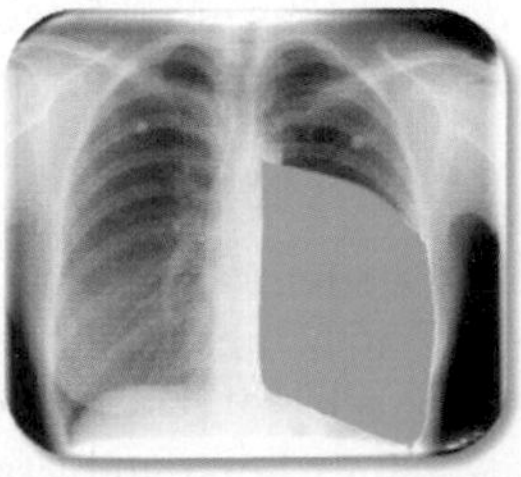	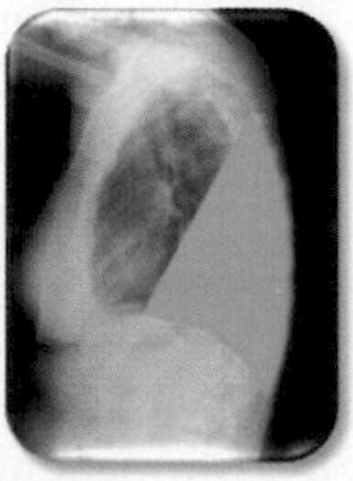

Fig. 5.2 Frontal and lateral views to illustrate the locations of the lung lobes in the thorax.

- The heart:
  - On a PA film the cardiac size should not exceed 50% of the thoracic diameter, termed the cardiothoracic ratio.

Table 5.2 Anatomy of the heart shadow on chest radiograph.

BORDER OF THE HEART ON PLAIN RADIOGRAPH	STRUCTURE
Right	Right atrium
Inferior	Right ventricle
Left	Left atrial appendage and left ventricle

MICRO-facts

On AP films, DO NOT comment on the size of the heart as it will always be magnified.

MICRO-facts

When presenting chest radiographs, try using the following approach.

- Film specifics
  - name
  - age
  - date of birth
  - ward
  - consultant.
- Technical factors
  - film projection, e.g. is the film AP? PA? Supine? Erect?
  - rotation: in a truly straight film, the spinous process lies equidistant from the medial heads of the clavicles
  - penetration: you should be able to see the vertebral bodies behind the heart
  - inspiration: to check for an adequate degree of inspiration, count the anterior ribs on the right. In a good radiograph, six anterior ribs should be visible above the right hemidiaphragm.
- View and comment on the
  - heart and major vessels
    - contour of heart and size

continued...

continued...

- lungs and pleura
  - symmetry
  - volume
  - vasculature
- mediastinum
  - hila
  - vasculature
  - paratracheal
- bones.
- Remember to pay particular attention to the review areas:
  - apices
  - hila
  - behind the heart
  - below the diaphragm
  - soft tissues (e.g. breast shadows) and bone.
- Offer a three- to four-line summary of the radiograph.
- Offer a differential diagnosis if possible.

COMMON FINDINGS ON PLAIN CHEST RADIOGRAPHS

Pneumothorax
- Erect film
  - Seen as a loss of lung markings between the lung and chest wall.
    - Magnification of digital films makes this sometimes subtle finding more obvious.
    - An expiration film may be useful for detection because the pneumothorax is likely to increase in size.
- Supine film
  - Lung edge may not be as visible.
  - Large, deep costophrenic sulcus may be evident.
  - Increased ipsilateral lucency of hemithorax and hemidiaphragm.
- If very large, pneumothorax may cause mediastinal shift = *tension pneumothorax.*
  - Mediastinal shift will be away from the side of the pneumothorax.
  - Needs immediate decompression – don't wait for a chest radiograph!
- Chronic chest diseases such as chronic obstructive pulmonary disease (COPD), asthma and cystic fibrosis all predispose to pneumothoraces.
- Smoking is also a risk factor.

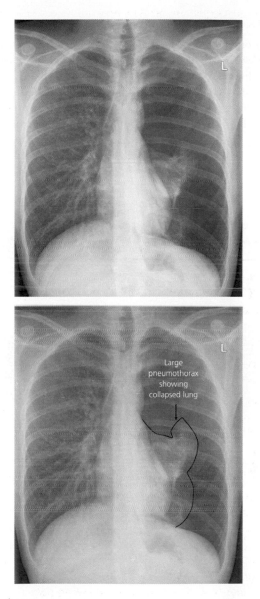

Fig. 5.3 Pneumothorax.

Pneumoperitoneum

- This is seen on an erect chest radiograph as free air under the diaphragm.
  - More evident under right hemi-diaphragm due to distinguishable upper liver border.
  - Harder to see under left hemi-diaphragm and not to be confused with gastric air (gastric bubble).
- Look for the following on the abdominal plain radiograph:
  - 'Rigler's sign' also known as 'double wall sign', is when air is present on both sides of the bowel wall;
  - falciform ligament sign – may outline the falciform ligament due to air on either side of it;

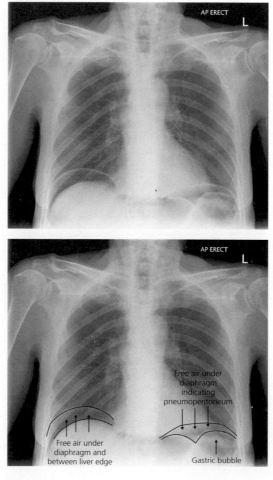

Fig. 5.4 Pneumoperitoneum.

- Beware of bowel loops below the diaphragm that can mimic pneumoperitoneum (Chilaiditi's sign).
- Causes include:
  - post-abdominal surgery/laparoscopy;
  - visceral perforation of the stomach or bowel;
  - perforated abscess/ulcer.

Lobar pneumonia

- With lobar pneumonia, there will be loss of the 'silhouette sign'.
  - The heart shadow and diaphragm are only seen if air is in the adjacent pulmonary acini.
  - Consolidation occurs in pneumonia, which obscures the silhouette.

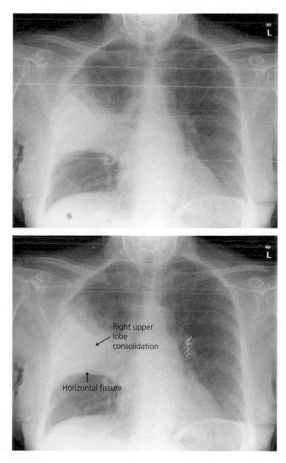

Fig. 5.5 Pneumonia.

Common clinical investigations

Table 5.3 Silhouettes and consolidation.

LUNG LOBE CONSOLIDATION	WHICH SILHOUETTE IS LOST
Right upper lobe	Right superior mediastinum
Right middle lobe	Right heart border
Right lower lobe	Right hemidiaphragm
Left upper lobe	Aortic knuckle
Left lower lobe	Left hemidiaphragm
Left lingual lobe	Left heart border

MICRO-facts

Remember that with lobar pneumonia, a 4–6 week follow-up chest radiograph is needed to ensure resolution of the pneumonia.

Pulmonary fibrosis

- This is seen as reticulonodular shadowing.
    - 'Lines and dots'.
    - Note that the cardiac and diaphragmatic silhouette may be visible.
    - In consolidation these may be obscured depending on the location of consolidation.
    - Cardiac shadow is described as a 'shaggy heart'.
- High-resolution CT scan is the gold standard of diagnosis.
- Fibrosis may be due to:
    - drugs (amiodarone, methotrexate);
    - rheumatoid arthritis;

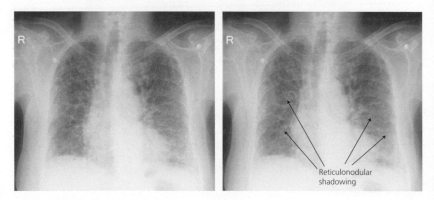

Reticulonodular shadowing

Fig. 5.6 Pulmonary fibrosis.

- ankylosing spondylitis;
- sarcoidosis;
- asbestosis;
- tuberculosis;
- extrinsic allergic alveolitis.

Left lower lobe collapse

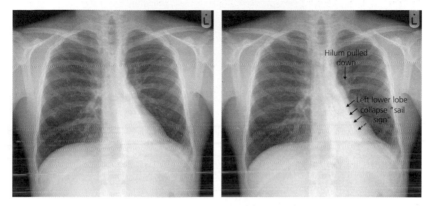

Hilum pulled
down

Left lower lobe
collapse "sail
sign"

Fig. 5.7 Lower lobe collapse.

- Look for the triangular appearance behind the left side of heart.
  - Left lower lobe collapses down behind heart = *'sail sign'*.
- Left hilum may also be pulled downwards due to the vacuumed pressure effect from the collapsed lung.

MICRO-facts

Any lung lobe may collapse. Features of pulmonary collapse include:
- increased opacification of involved lobe
- volume loss of hemithorax due to collapsed lobe
  - tracheal or hilar shift;
  - elevation of hemidiaphragm;
  - shift of mediastinum or fissures.
- compensatory hyperinflation of surrounding lung lobes
- loss of volume of collapsed lobe:
  - crowding of ribs;
  - displacement of the hila or fissures towards collapsed lobe;
  - mediastinal shift towards collapsed lobe.

Common clinical investigations

Left upper lobe collapse

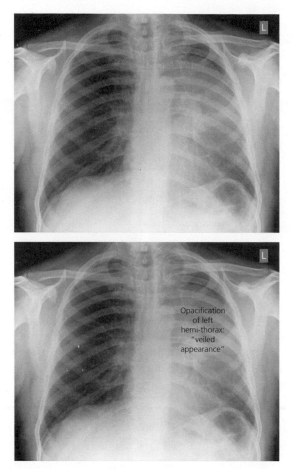

Opacification
of left
hemi-thorax:
"veiled
appearance"

Fig. 5.8 Left upper lobe collapse.

- Look for:
    - diffuse opacification ('veiled appearance') of the left hemithorax;
    - left upper lobe collapsed anteriorly to give this appearance;
    - decreased visibility of the aortic knuckle and left heart border;
    - diaphragmatic elevation;
    - the underlying cause, typically a hilar mass.

Congestive cardiac failure

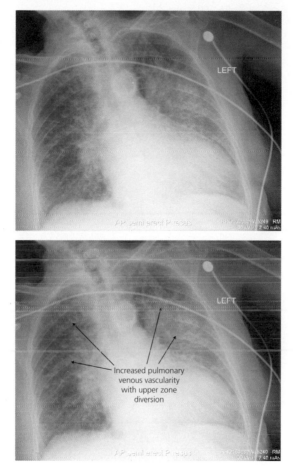

Fig. 5.9 Congestive cardiac failure (AP projection).

- Look for the 'ABCDE' signs:
    - **A** – **A**lveolar bat wings;
    - **B** – Kerley **B** lines (1–2 cm long horizontal lines perpendicular to the pleural surface of fluid-filled fissures intralobular septal at the costophrenic angles);
    - **C** – **C**ardiomegaly (indicating enlarged left ventricle);
    - **D** – upper lobe **D**iversion (arteriolar vasoconstriction due to alveolar hypoxia);
    - **E** – pleural **E**ffusions (seen as a meniscus sign on an erect radiograph. On a supine radiograph, look for ill-defined, opacification with pulmonary vessels still visible).

Common clinical investigations

Emphysema

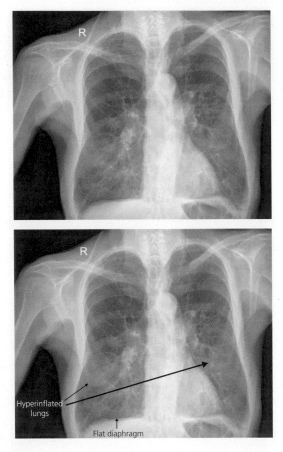

Fig. 5.10 Emphysema.

- Look for
  - barrel-shaped lung fields signifying hyperinflated lungs
    – greater than 10 ribs visible posteriorly
  - flattened hemidiaphragms
  - enlarged central pulmonary arteries (attenuated vasculature)
  - peripheral pruning
  - horizontal ribs
  - bullae (air pockets).
- Often seen in patients with COPD.

Tuberculosis (TB)

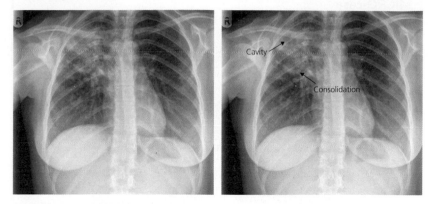

Fig. 5.11 Tuberculosis.

- Tuberculosis may form:
  - ill-defined nodular opacities with cavitation;
  - pleural thickening;
  - fibrocalcific change, usually in the upper lobes;
  - pericardial effusions;
  - miliary shadowing;
  - pleural calcification.

MICRO-facts

Note that if TB is suspected, the patient should be isolated immediately, with appropriate barrier nursing.

- Note there are many causes of a cavitating lung lesion on a plain radiograph. These include:
  - TB;
  - lung tumour/metastases;
  - cavitating pneumonia;
  - lung abscess;
  - lung infarction;
  - vasculitic disease such as Wegener's granulomatosis.

Common clinical investigations

MICRO-case

Note that when interpreting radiographs, do not instantly stop once you think you have spotted the abnormality. There may be more than one thing to see. Interpret the radiograph below.

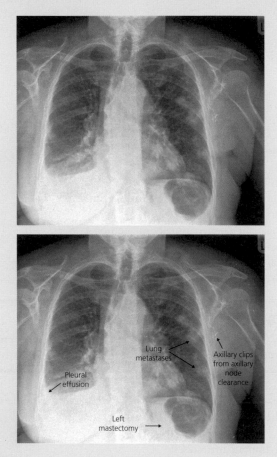

Fig. 5.12 Micro-case 1.

This radiograph shows multiple diffuse nodules bilaterally. But don't stop here! On further inspection, you may notice that the patient is a female with only the right breast shadow present, and there is also evidence of surgical staples in the left axilla. These signs both point to the fact that the patient has had a mastectomy with axillary node clearance, and hence it is likely that this patient has been surgically treated for breast cancer. This radiograph is showing metastatic spread to the lungs from her breast cancer, with signs of a right-sided pleural effusion.

Common clinical investigations

COMMON FINDINGS ON PLAIN ABDOMINAL RADIOGRAPHS

- Plain abdominal radiographs are rarely helpful and should never be 'routine' in non-specific acute abdominal pain.
- Their use should be reserved exclusively for cases where clinical suspicion is high for the few conditions that may be diagnosed with the test, e.g.:
  - renal/ureteric calculi;
  - small/large bowel obstruction, including volvulus;
  - bowel perforation and pneumoperitoneum;
  - colitis.

MICRO-facts

When presenting an abdominal radiograph, try using the following approach.

- Film specifics
  - name
  - age
  - date of birth
  - ward
  - consultant.
- Technical factors
  - Is the whole abdomen in view?
    - Can you see the diaphragm above?
    - Can you see the hernial orifices below?
  - Is there adequate penetration?
- Explain what you can see
  - Look for and comment on any lines/tubes/wires/artefacts.
  - Look at the bowel calibre, distribution and gas pattern.
  - Look at the soft tissues, including the hollow and solid organs. These may include the:
    - solid organs: liver, spleen, pancreas and kidneys;
    - hollow organs: stomach, bladder, bowel, uterus and gallbladder.
  - Look at the bones and any other visible calcification
    - Note that "normal" calcifications include: costal cartilages; aorta; iliac arteries; splenic artery; pelvic phleboliths; fibroids; mesenteric lymph nodes.
    - Note that abnormal calcification may include: renal tract calculi; aneurysms; gallbladder wall; pancreatitis; appendicolith.
- Remember to pay particular attention to the review areas:
  - lung bases (if shown)
  - line of ureters (for calculi)
  - hernial orifices.
- Offer a three- to four-line summary of the radiograph.
- Offer a differential diagnosis if possible.

Common clinical investigations

Renal stone disease

- Up to 60% of calculi may be seen on a KUB (kidneys, ureter and bladder) radiograph.
- Look for calculi as an increased focal opacification in the distribution of:
  - the kidney;
  - along the route of the ureter – adjacent to the medial border of the psoas muscle, along the transverse processes of the spine;
  - the bladder.
- The gold standard in identifying calculi and the level of ureteric obstruction is a **computed tomography (CT)-KUB** $\pm$ CT-intravenous urogram (IVU).
  - CT-KUB is the first-line investigation conducted with suspected calculi, which may also detect other pathologies, such as an abdominal aortic aneurysm. This is a non-contrast scan.
  - A KUB radiograph is then taken as a method of follow-up once the location of a calculus has been identified on CT (assuming it is radio-opaque).
  - If the calculus is not radio-opaque on a KUB, then follow-up is conducted using CT.
  - If the IVU component is performed, look for an enhanced nephrogram, delayed excretion, hydronephrosis, hydroureter and standing column.

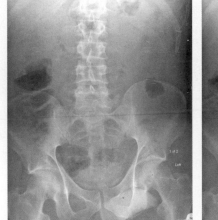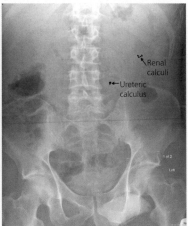

Fig. 5.13 Ureteric calculus.

Small bowel obstruction

- Look for:
    - central bowel loops with variable amounts of fluid and gas;
    - gas may not be see in small bowel if the loops are fluid-filled;
    - valvulae conniventes across the lumen of the bowel. Maximum normal diameter of the small bowel is 3 cm;
    - collapse of the large bowel loops.
- Note that the more distal the obstruction, the more small bowel loops visible.
- Small bowel obstruction may be due to:
    - adhesions (e.g. post-operative);
    - hernias;
    - tumours;
    - gallstone ileus;
    - volvulus;
    - intussusception;
    - congenital atresia (babies).
- CT scans should be performed in all patients with suspected small bowel obstruction, in an attempt to identify the cause and location of obstruction, along with assessment for perforation.

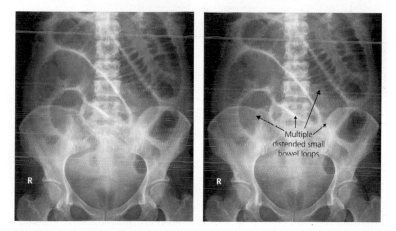

Fig. 5.14 Small bowel obstruction.

Large bowel obstruction

- Look for:
    - peripheral bowel loops;
    - haustral markings of the bowel loops;
    - maximum normal diameter of bowel is 5.5 cm (caecum up to 8 cm),
    - the cut-off point, which may be visible.

Common clinical investigations

- Note that in suspected large bowel obstruction, CT is the investigation of choice after a plain radiograph, in order to identify the location and cause of obstruction, along with any sign of perforation.
- Note that large bowel obstruction is very susceptible to perforation, especially if the ileocaecal valve is competent as it prevents decompression of the dilated caecum into the distal ileum.
- Causes of large bowel obstruction include:
    - tumours;
    - complicated diverticular disease;
    - volvulus;
    - hernias.

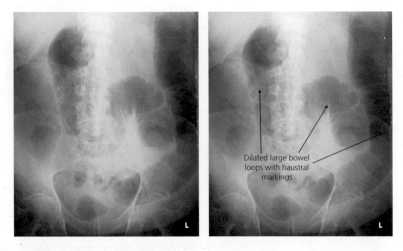

Fig. 5.15 Large bowel obstruction.

Colitis

- Features of severe colitis include:
    - thickening/oedema of the colonic wall ('thumbprinting' sign);
    - thickening/loss of haustrations.
- In advanced cases, there may be intramural air, portal venous gas and a pneumoperitoneum (especially in neonates).
- Colitis may occur in the following:
    - inflammatory bowel disease;
    - pseudomembranous colitis (*Clostridium difficile* infection);
    - ischaemic bowel.
- A plain radiograph will not identify the cause of colitis, so other investigations with respect to the patient's symptoms will contribute to reaching the diagnosis.

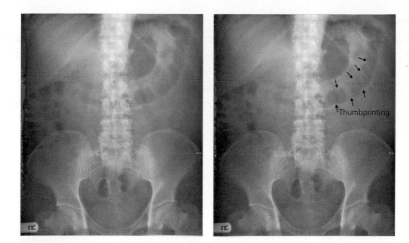

Fig. 5.16 Colitis.

Sigmoid volvulus

- This obstructs bowel transit and hence presents as a large bowel obstruction.
- Characteristically there is a 'coffee bean' sign on the left side, with the absence of haustrations in the affected part of bowel.
- Note that the caecum is usually visible and dilated in the right lower quadrant, distinguishing it radiologically from a caecal volvulus.

> **MICRO-print**
> On a water-soluble enema, the sigmoid volvulus will show a 'bird's beak' sign at the site of the obstruction.

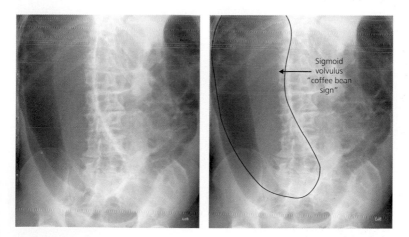

Fig. 5.17 Sigmoid volvulus.

Common clinical investigations

Caecal volvulus

- This obstructs the terminal ileum, and therefore presents as a small bowel obstruction.
- The gas-filled caecum will come to lie ectopically in the left or right hypochondrium, rather than the right iliac fossa (known as the 'empty caecum sign').
- Distal to the volvulus, the large bowel will be empty and devoid of air.
- There is a risk of perforation as a result of the enlarging caecal dilatation.

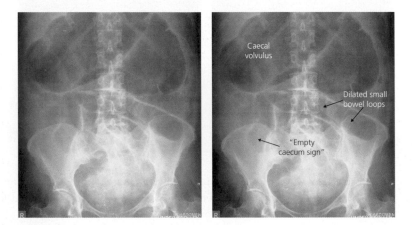

Fig. 5.18 Caecal volvulus.

MICRO-case

Here is a model example of how to present an abdominal plain radiograph. Try presenting it yourself before reading the example:

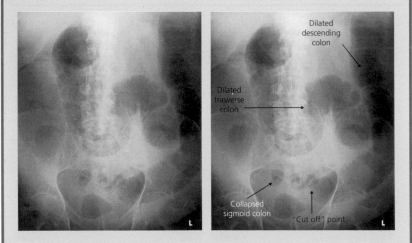

Fig. 5.19 Micro-case 2.

continued...

continued...

Patient details
    Name: Mrs Humpty Dumpty
    DOB: 24/7/61
    Hospital number: 4875933
    Date radiograph taken: 2/3/11
    Ward: F4
    Consultant: Mr Farrow

This is a frontal abdominal radiograph. The radiograph was taken with adequate penetration but inadequate coverage as the diaphragm is not in view superiorly, and the hernial orifices are not entirely visible inferiorly.

On general inspection, there are no signs of artefact or foreign materials. On inspection of the bowel, I cannot see any small bowel markings, and the large bowel seems to be dilated from the point of the hepatic flexure, with haustrations visible on the transverse, descending and sigmoid colon. The remaining soft-tissue organs with the abdomen appear normal. On inspection of the bony structures, I would suspect an element of osteoarthritis in the right hip joint due to evidence of joint space narrowing, which would need to be further assessed by an adequate hip joint radiograph. There is no evidence of any calcification.

In summary, this is a plain abdominal radiograph of a 49-year-old woman with dilated large bowel. This is in keeping with a diagnosis of large bowel obstruction at the level of the sigmoid colon.

COMMON FINDINGS ON PLAIN MUSCULOSKELETAL RADIOGRAPHS

MICRO-facts

When presenting a musculoskeletal radiograph, try using the following approach.

- Film specifics
    - name
    - age
    - date of birth
    - ward
    - consultant

continued...

continued...

- Technical factors
  - What projection do you have?
  - Would you like more than one projection?
    - Two views, taken at 90°, should be performed in cases of trauma
    - This ensures any fractures are not missed.
- Clinical history
  - Read this thoroughly.
- Comment on what you can see:
  - periarticular calcification
  - bone texture and architecture
  - bone alignment and cortex
  - joint spaces
  - soft tissue.
- Remember to declare any foreign body evident and compare sides if possible.
- Note that when describing any fractures, comment on:
  - open or closed fracture?
  - general site: proximal/mid/distal
  - fracture line: transverse/oblique/spiral/segmental/greenstick?
  - comminution/impaction/intra-articular?
  - resulting position:
    - deformity? stable/unstable?
    - angulation? displacement?
    - rotation.

Hip fracture

- Look for whether the fracture is intracapsular or extracapsular.
  - Intracapsular – the fracture is between the blood supply and the head of the femur; resulting in a risk of avascular necrosis.
  - Intracapsular fractures may be subdivided into whether they are:
    - displaced;
    - undisplaced.
  - Extracapsular – is where the head of the femur maintains its blood supply.
  - Extracapsular fractures comprise intertrochanteric and subtrochanteric fractures, and are often treated with internal fixation (dynamic hip screw).

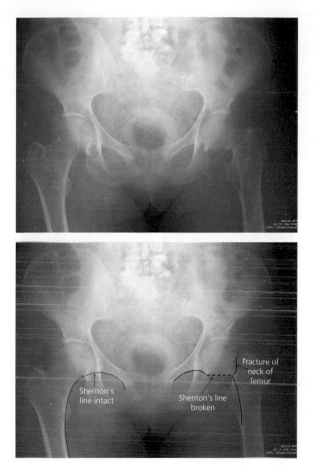

Fig. 5.20 Hip fracture.

Common clinical investigations

MICRO-print

Note that hip fractures are often classified by the **Garden classification** which relies only upon the appearance of the hip on the AP radiograph. It is used to determine the appropriate treatment, according to the risk of avascular necrosis:

- **Garden stage I**: undisplaced incomplete fracture, which includes valgus impacted fractures.
- **Garden stage II**: undisplaced, complete fractures.
- **Garden stage III**: complete fracture, which is partially displaced.
- **Garden stage IV**: complete fracture, which is completely displaced.

MICRO-facts

Note that when reviewing a hip radiograph, it is useful to delineate *Shenton's line* as an interruption in this line can indicate a fractured neck of femur or a developmental dysplasia of the hip, given an appropriate clinical scenario. Shenton's line is an imaginary line drawn along the inferior border of the superior pubic ramus (superior border of the obturator foramen) and along the inferomedial border of the neck of the femur. This line should be smooth and continuous.

Colles' fracture

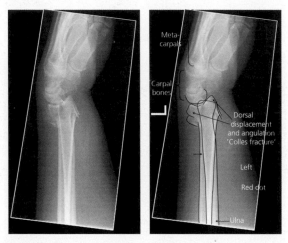

Fig. 5.21 Colles' fracture.

- Common injury in middle-aged to older people due to a fall on an outstretched hand (FOOSH).
- Look for:
  - fracture of distal radius, with dorsal angulation on a lateral view, giving a 'dinner fork deformity';
  - shortening of the distal radius may occur, resulting in radial angulation of the hand/wrist;
  - associated fractures:
    - ulnar styloid – no treatment needed;
    - scaphoid fracture.

Greenstick fracture (or Torus)

- A fracture of any long bone, e.g. ulna, radius, tibia in the paediatric population.

- An incomplete fracture in which there is a buckle or kink in the bone cortex on the convex side, but with complete continuity of the cortex on the other side.
- Occurs as a result of angular force.
- May be associated with deformity and hence easy to detect.

Smith's fracture

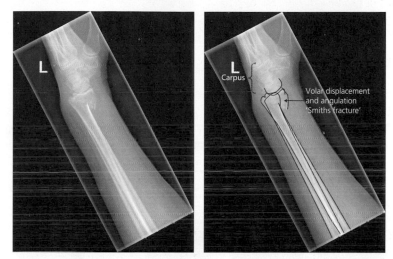

Fig. 5.22 Smith's fracture.

- Often the result of a fall on a flexed wrist and is the opposite of a Colles' fracture (sometimes referred to as a reversed Colles').
- Look for a fracture of the distal radius, with anterior angulation (also known as volar/palmar displacement) of the hand/wrist.
- Note that this requires referral to an orthopaedic surgeon as it is normally treated with internal fixation as a plaster cast often results in malunion and poor function.

Scaphoid fracture

- Most common carpal bone to fracture.
- Suspected when there is tenderness in the anatomical snuff box.
- In suspected scaphoid fracture, ensure a four-view, 'scaphoid series' is requested.
    - This includes two oblique views, one AP view and one lateral view.
- Often no fracture will be seen on the initial radiograph, and radiographs are repeated in 10–14 days.

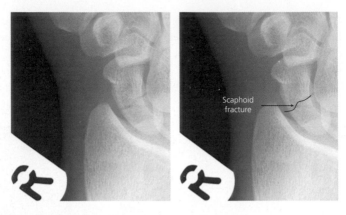

Fig. 5.23 Scaphoid fracture.

- Patients should initially be treated as if they have a scaphoid fracture even if one is not seen, to avoid complications such as:
    - avascular necrosis of the proximal fragment;
    - non-union.

Gout

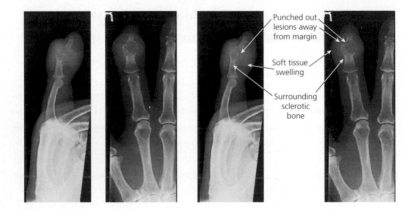

Fig. 5.24 Gout.

- Initial radiographs may be normal.
- Recurrent gout in a joint may lead to the following radiological features:
    - 'punched out' erosions away from the joint margin;
    - soft-tissue swelling;
    - surrounding sclerotic bone;
    - joint space preservation;
    - tophaceous deposits in the periarticular soft tissues.

Osteoarthritis

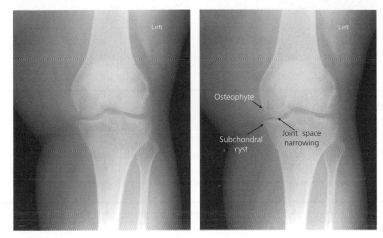

Fig. 5.25 Osteoarthritis.

- There are four signs on a radiograph of osteoarthritis:
  - joint space narrowing (non-uniform);
  - subchondral bone cysts;
  - osteophyte formation;
  - subchondral sclerosis;
- Note the asymmetrical nature of osteoarthritis.
- Remember:
  - in the hands, the first carpal, metacarpal and interphalangeal joints are most commonly affected;
  - in the feet, the first metatarsophalangeal joint is most commonly affected.

MICRO-facts

Remember that patients with rheumatoid arthritis may also have cervical spine involvement, and so if any patient with rheumatoid arthritis requires a general anaesthetic, then a lateral flexion plain radiograph of the neck should be taken to allow appropriate precautions to be taken during intubation.

Rheumatoid arthritis

- Look for the following features on a hand radiograph:
  - Soft-tissue swelling;
  - periarticular osteopenia;
  - bony erosions;
  - joint space narrowing centred on the metacarpophalangeal joints;

Common clinical investigations

- sparing of the distal interphalangeal joints;
- ulnar deviation;
- swan-neck deformity;
- Boutonnière deformity;
- pannus formation (granular inflammation).

MICRO-print

- Note that in rheumatoid arthritis, the distal interphalangeal joints are spared as they do not contain any synovium.
- Also of interest is the periarticular osteopenia, which is due to the infiltration and pooling of cytokines, which leads to bone resorption. This is in contrast to the subchondral sclerosis found in osteoarthritis.

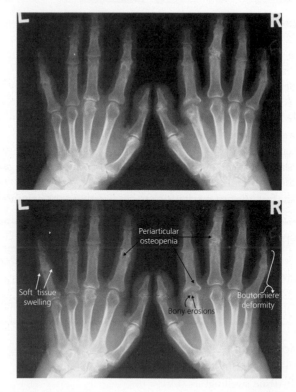

Fig. 5.26 Rheumatoid arthritis.

5.2 BASICS OF ULTRASOUND SCANS

Fig. 5.27 is a sample image of an ultrasound of a patient with appendicitis.

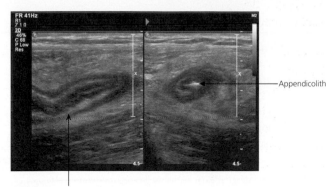

Fig. 5.27 Ultrasound scan.

WHAT ARE ULTRASOUND SCANS?

- Ultrasound waves produced by an electromagnetic field are emitted through a probe, and reflected back by tissues to be detected by the same probe.
- This is then projected on a monitor, and the echogenicity of structures is distinguished by different shades of grey.
- Different probes with different frequency wave emissions are available depending on the structures being imaged.
- Fatty tissue is slightly brighter (hyperechoic) than surrounding tissue.
- The Doppler effect can allow movement of blood to be detected with the use of sound waves.

INDICATIONS

- Examples using ultrasound waves:
  - cardiac imaging (ECHO), imaging of thoracic, abdominal and genitourinary organs, along with anatomical detail of joints;
  - this also allows visualization for invasive procedures to be carried out such as chest drain insertion, or ultrasound-guided biopsies.
- Examples using Doppler ultrasound:
  - peripheral vascular disease;
  - deep vein thrombosis;
  - venous insufficiency;
  - portal hypertension;
  - fetal maternal imaging of umbilical blood flow;
  - portal or hepatic vein thrombosis.

Common clinical investigations

PREPARATIONS

- Patients undergoing hepatobiliary ultrasound should be fasted for at least 6 hours.
- Patients undergoing pelvic ultrasound should have a full bladder.

ADVANTAGES AND DISADVANTAGES

- No ionizing radiation.
- Portable machine available.
- Images are instantaneous and in real time.
- Ultrasound waves cannot penetrate gas or bone, so overlying ribs and aerated lung restrict imaging of the deep thoracic structures or bowel gas obscuring the pancreas or aorta.
- Difficult to image subjects who have excessive overlying tissue, e.g. obese patients.
- Difficult to analyse retrospective images when the location of the transducer probe is unknown.
- May be operator dependent.

5.3 BASICS OF COMPUTED TOMOGRAPHY

WHAT IS COMPUTED TOMOGRAPHY?

- A series of two-dimensional images, representing sections through the body, thickness varying from < 1–10 mm, which when put together can form a three-dimensional image.
- Uses X-ray technology which rotates in a tube around the patient while emitting a beam through the patient, allowing precise differentiation between tissue densities.

INDICATIONS

- Any area may be scanned for anatomical detail/pathology.
- To allow assessment when planning radiotherapy.
- Staging of tumours (to assess potential for operative cure, or for chemotherapy baseline assessment) and follow up response to treatment.

ADVANTAGES

- Allows detailed assessment of a patient's anatomy, especially internal organs.
- Oral contrast may be used to outline the gastrointestinal tract.
- IV contrast may be used, outlining the vascular system or organs.
- Fast to perform, e.g. the chest may be imaged in a single breath-hold.
- Available for emergency or elective requests, depending on the clinical scenario.
- Good images obtained in obese patients (unlike ultrasound) as fat separates the abdominal organs.

DISADVANTAGES

- It is relatively expensive.
- A high dose of ionizing radiation is required.
- The machine lacks portability.
- There is a small, but real, risk of anaphylaxis when contrast agents used.

INTERPRETATION

- Orientation:
    - CT images are usually viewed in the horizontal (**axial**) plane.
    - Conventionally, all **axial** images are viewed as if looking upward from the feet of the patient towards the head.
    - Therefore, the organs on the right side of the patient are on the left side of the image and *vice versa*.
    - **Coronal** images are vertical slices through the body from front to back.
    - **Sagittal** images are vertical slices through the body from the left hand side of the body to the right or *vice versa*.
- Attenuation:
    - Images on CT on a 'greyscale', depending on their density, and hence the amount of radiation they absorb.
    - Attenuation is the process by which a beam of radiation is reduced in intensity when passing through material.
    - Low-attenuation tissue suggests it is relatively transparent (e.g. air), but on CT will appear dark.
    - High-attenuation tissue is a denser material (e.g. bone) and will appear brighter on CT.
- Hounsfield units (HU):
    - These are the units of X-ray attenuation.
    - Each tissue has a specific unit, depending on how bright or dark it appears (the brighter the tissue, the higher the HU): bone, $+1000$; water, 0; air, -1000.
    - Bone will therefore appear white.
    - Blood contains protein making it dense, and areas of acute bleeding appear highly attenuated (bright) on CT.
    - Areas of dead or damaged brain tissue will become less dense, meaning that they will appear darker (lower attenuation), for example an established infarct in relation to the surrounding brain.

CT scans are reported by specialists. Their detailed interpretation is therefore beyond the scope of this book. We have, however, included case studies to illustrate some key points, given that clinicians view CT images in the context of multidisciplinary and clinical radiology meetings.

Common clinical investigations

MICRO-cases

MICRO-case 3. An 84-year-old male nursing home resident presents with increasing drowsiness. The care assistant who attended with him informs you he has become increasingly unsteady and confused over the past 2 weeks since falling in the bathroom and has deteriorated rapidly over the past 24 hours. A CT scan was performed (Fig. 5.28).

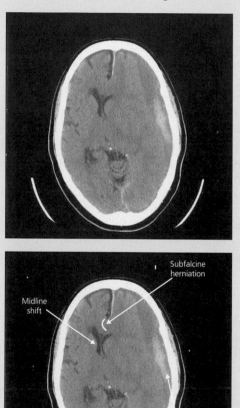

Fig. 5.28 Micro-case 3.

On reporting this CT scan, it is evident that this is a left-sided low-density subdural collection with an area of high density within. There is also visible midline shift to the right with effacement of sulci and the left lateral ventricle. This is all in keeping with an acute on chronic subdural haemorrhage.

continued...

continued...

Learning points
- Fresh blood is denser on CT than older areas of bleeding (see Chapter 10, Neurology).
- Note the characteristic differences between a subdural and extradural haemorrhage:

	Extradural	Subdural
Source of blood	Middle meningeal artery	Dural veins
Size	Small – limited by skull vaults	Large
Shape	Convex 'coconut'	Concave 'banana'
Crosses sutures?	Cannot cross sutures	Can cross sutures
Crosses midline?	May cross midline	Does not cross midline
Position related to injury	Directly adjacent to injury site	Often distant from injury site – contre coup
Attenuation	High attenuation	High attenuation in acute phase, can also be low (chronic) or mixed attenuation (acute on chronic)

MICRO-case 4. A car travelling at approximately 25 mph hits a 20-year-old pedestrian. He is thrown to the ground some distance away by the impact and sustains multiple injuries, including a head injury. Upon arrival at A&E his GCS is 13/15. CT scan is shown in Fig. 5.29, using the bone window filters.

On reporting this scan, a depressed skull fracture can be seen in the right parietal bone, with associated soft-tissue swelling.

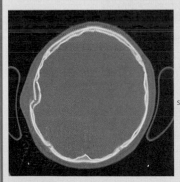 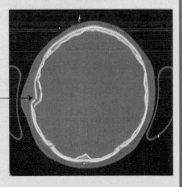

Depressed skin fracture →

Fig. 5.29 Micro-case 4.

continued...

Common clinical investigations

continued...

Learning points

- In young children, the suture lines may not have fully fused and so a suture may be mistaken for a fracture line. They may however be distinguished by the fact that sutures are not as straight as fracture lines.
- Note that this image is seen in the bone window filter. Once a CT scan has been acquired, the parameters of the greyscale can be manipulated to favour the viewing of certain structures.
- Depending on their density, their Hounsfield unit can be specified so that the image only views structures within the image that are of the specified Hounsfield unit. In this case, the Hounsfield unit of bone (+1000) has been specified, making an accurate assessment of the brain parenchyma impossible.

MICRO-case 5. This 59-year-old man is experiencing severe left-sided flank pain, which he describes as colicky and intermittent. The patient is also complaining of nausea and vomiting. He therefore attended A&E this morning. He is known to have an abdominal aortic aneurysm (AAA). A CT scan was performed (Fig. 5.30).

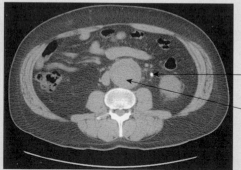

Midureteric calculus

AAA

Fig. 5.30 Micro-case 5.

This CT scan shows a proximal ureteric stone in his left ureter (high attenuation). The abdominal aorta is enlarged – visible anterior to the vertebral body.

Learning points

- CT-KUB is an extremely sensitive investigation for locating renal stones.
- Locating the calculus on CT may make it easier to identify it on plain KUB radiographs. Progress of the stone through the urinary tract may then be monitored.
- Clinical presentation of ruptured AAA and ureteric stones may be similar, therefore non-contrast CT is an ideal test to investigate both pathologies.

5.4 BASICS OF MAGNETIC RESONANCE IMAGING

WHAT IS MAGNETIC RESONANCE IMAGING?

- Protons within the nucleus of a hydrogen atom spin and align within a magnetic field. A radiofrequency (RF) pulse applied upon the magnetic field at $90°$ changes the alignment of the protons.
- Once the RF pulse stops, the protons shed their new energy to their surroundings (T_1 relaxation) – giving a T_1-weighted image. Thereafter, the protons stop spinning (T_2 relaxation), giving a T_2-weighted image.
- T_1-weighted images provide good anatomical detail.
- T_2-weighted images provide good detail of tissue pathology.
- Many other sequences may be performed.

INDICATIONS

- Magnetic resonance imaging (MRI) provides high quality, accurate imaging of the central nervous system, musculoskeletal system, heart, central and peripheral vascular systems (magnetic resonance angiography (MRA)), abdominal organs including biliary tree (magnetic resonance cholangiopancreatography (MRCP)) and pelvic organs.
- It allows local staging of some neoplasms, such as rectal, bladder and prostate.

CONTRAINDICATIONS

- Pacemakers and cochlear implant.
- Ferromagnetic foreign bodies in eye.
- Some arterial aneurysm clips.

ADVANTAGES

- No ionizing radiation.
- Excellent anatomical detail, especially soft-tissue differentiation.
- Images in axial, sagittal and coronal planes without reconstruction of images (unlike CT).

DISADVANTAGES

- Expensive.
- Time taken to acquire image is longer than CT.
- Lungs give poor image quality.
- Calcification imaged with poor accuracy.
- Patients must remain very still throughout the procedure, therefore not suitable for children or very unwell patients, unless sedated/anaesthetized.

Common clinical investigations

- Confined space is claustrophobic.
- Noisy inside the scanner for patients.

MRI scans are reported by specialists. Their detailed interpretation is therefore beyond the scope of this book. However, we have included case studies below to illustrate some key points.

MICRO-facts

At the early stage in your career, it is far more important to understand the indications for MRI scanning, than how to interpret them.

MICRO-cases

MICRO-case 6. This 33-year-old woman has had intermittent episodes of numbness and tingling of the limbs, ataxia, visual disturbances, and episodes of facial paraesthesia. All the above symptoms developed spontaneously, followed by periods of improvement for a few months in between. She was therefore referred to the neurologists, who considered multiple sclerosis within their differential diagnosis. After having conducted the relevant blood tests and CSF analysis, a MRI scan was conducted (Fig. 5.31).

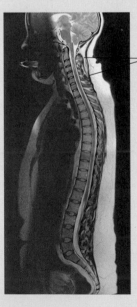

High signal change in the spinal cord, in keeping with demyelination

Fig. 5.31 Micro-case 6.

continued...

continued...

The above T_2 sequence shows the CSF as high signal (white). Within the spinal cord at the levels of C1–C3, areas of high signal are present, in keeping with demyelination plaques.

Learning points

- MRI is the investigation of choice in multiple sclerosis, confirming the diagnosis by demonstrating the presence of high signal plaques, which represent areas of demyelination.
- These are found in the periventicular deep white matter on a T_2-weighted sequence, and may be seen throughout the central nervous system, including the spinal cord, brainstem and optic nerves.

MICRO-case 7. This 38-year-old man experienced acute-onset shooting pain into his leg associated with low back pain. Upon referral, an urgent MRI scan was requested (Fig. 5.32).

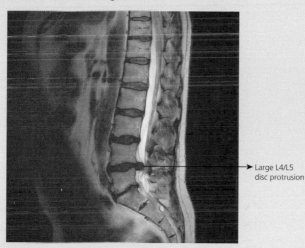

Large L4/L5
disc protrusion

Fig. 5.32 Micro-case 7.

Learning points

- Plain radiographs do have a role in imaging spinal disorders, such as in spinal trauma; however, the value of plain radiographs in back pain is questionable, because the spinal cord and nerves are not visible on these images.
- MRI, however, allows visualization of the vertebrae, spinal canal and its contents, making it the prefered investigation for degenerative, inflammatory and malignant conditions.
- The MRI T_2-weighted image in **Fig. 5.32** shows disc herniation into the spinal canal, between L4 and L5 vertebrae. On a T_1-weighted MRI scan, fat appears as high signal, while CSF and intervertebral discs are of low signal
- Note that 95% of disc protrusions occur in the two lowest spaces, L4–L5 or L5–S1.

Part II

Clinical specialties

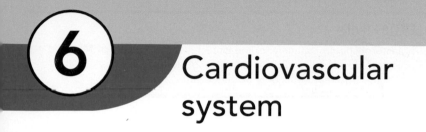

6 Cardiovascular system

6.1 BLOOD TESTS

BASIC BLOOD TESTS

- Full blood count:
  - Chronic anaemia may precipitate cardiac failure, or cause angina due to hypoperfusion.
  - Leucocytosis secondary to infection may exacerbate cardiac failure.
  - A neutophilia is common post myocardial infarction (MI) due to myocardial necrosis.
- Urea and electrolytes (U + E):
  - In cardiogenic shock renal function may become impaired.
  - Drugs including angiotensin-converting enzyme (ACE) inhibitors and diuretics can negatively affect renal function, e.g. hypokalaemia and hyponatraemia are common with diuretic therapy.
  - Electrolyte disturbances may predispose to arrhythmias, e.g. tachyarrhythmias in hyperkalaemia.
- Liver function tests:
  - Liver congestion from right heart failure may lead to impaired hepatic function and elevate hepatic enzymes.
  - Can be deranged by alcohol intake, which may be a cause of arrhythmias or cardiomyopathy.
- Arterial blood gases:
  - May show hypoxia, hypercapnia and respiratory acidosis in patients with cardiac failure.
- Thyroid function tests:
  - Low thyroid hormone may be a cause of a sinus bradycardia.
  - Thyrotoxicosis is a cause of atrial fibrillation and tachycardia, and may lead to cardiac failure if left untreated.
- Blood lipid profile:
  - Hyperlipidaemia may predispose to hypertension and ischaemic heart disease.
  - Hypercholesterolaemia is a risk factor for MI.

> ## MICRO-facts
> Cholesterol should routinely be measured within 24 hours of MI.
> Cholesterol levels fall artificially low after 24 hours post MI. After this
> period, the true reading is only obtained after 2 months.

- Blood cultures:
  - If endocarditis is suspected, at least three sets should be sent within a
    24 hour period, each from a different site. Ideally, this should be done
    prior to antibiotic therapy, but this would depend on the severity of
    illness.
- Erythrocyte sedimentation rate and C-reactive protein:
  - These are markers of inflammation and infection and are useful for
    assessment of infective endocarditis and vasculitis.
- Brain natriuretic peptide:
  - This increases water excretion and causes peripheral vasodilatation,
    therefore reducing cardiac load.
  - Increased levels in cardiac failure are a homeostatic measure to protect
    the heart.

ASSESSMENT OF ACUTE CORONARY SYNDROMES

- Acute coronary syndromes form a spectrum of coronary artery disease
  varying from mild to acutely life-threatening conditions.
- All are due to narrowing of the coronary arteries due to atherosclerosis.
- Angina:
  - Exertion-induced ischaemia and chest pain due to coronary stenosis,
    which always resolves with rest.
- Unstable angina, non-ST segment elevation myocardial infarction (NSTEMI)
  and ST segment elevation myocardial infarction (STEMI):
  - These are due to rupture of atherosclerotic plaques within the
    coronaries.
  - Unstable angina causes temporary ischaemia which does not lead to
    myocardial damage.
  - In NSTEMI, there is myocardial damage without full-thickness
    infarction of the myocardium.
  - In STEMI, there is myocardial damage which, if left untreated, may
    progress to full-thickness infarction of the myocardium.
- An electrocardiogram (ECG) should be performed in all cases of chest pain
  to differentiate these conditions (see later under Electrocardiography, 6.2)
- Troponin assays should then be employed to differentiate unstable angina
  from NSTEMI (see Table 6.1).

Table 6.1 Differential diagnosis of acute coronary syndromes.

ACUTE CORONARY SYNDROME	ECG FINDINGS	TROPONIN ASSAY
Angina	None or features of ischaemia: T-wave inversion or ST segment depression	Negative
Unstable angina	None or features of ischaemia: T-wave inversion or ST segment depression	Negative
Non-ST-segment myocardial infarction	None or features of ischaemia: T-wave inversion or ST-segment depression	Positive
ST-elevation myocardial infarction	ST segment elevation	Positive

CARDIAC ENZYME BLOOD TESTS: INDICATORS OF MYOCARDIAL DAMAGE

- Troponin T and troponin I:
  - Enzymes highly specific to myocardial cells.
  - The gold standard blood test in suspected acute coronary syndrome (ACS).

MICRO-facts

In cases of high clinical suspicion of ACS, treatment should be based on clinical grounds as patients may present before troponin levels have risen.

MICRO-facts

Many other cardiovascular (e.g. myopericarditis, cardiac failure, pulmonary emboli, tachycardia, e.g. fast atrial fibrillation) and non-cardiovascular conditions (e.g. renal failure) may also elevate troponin levels; therefore, always interpret the result in the context of the overall clinical picture.

- Serum levels rise within 6–14 hours of the onset of a NSTEMI or STEMI and remain elevated for up to 14 days.
- Generally the troponin level is taken 12 hours after the onset of symptoms.
  - A negative troponin level at 12 hours after the worst chest pain is highly accurate in excluding myocardial damage.
- Any detectable troponin level indicates myocardial damage and confers an increased risk of mortality/morbidity regardless of the cause.

- Troponin levels at 6 hours after the onset of symptoms are sometimes taken in high clinical suspicion of MI, and if elevated may guide immediate treatment.
- Some emergency departments take a sample for troponin on admission to the unit, regardless of timescale.
  - A positive result at that point may lead to immediate treatment.
  - Further rises may be compared with a baseline level.
- Care is needed for interpretation of the test.
  - A positive result within an appropriate timeframe is diagnostic of acute myocardial infarction **only** in the appropriate clinical context.
  - Any cause of myocardial damage, e.g. myopericarditis, pulmonary embolism (due to backflow pressure), tachycardia (e.g. fast atrial fibrillation) or hypovolaemia may elevate troponin levels.
  - **Clinical assessment is therefore of paramount importance** to differentiate these causes from coronary artery pathology.
- An ECG is the most important initial investigation in suspected ACS.

MICRO-facts

Newer, 'high sensitivity' assays are being used in some centres which detect troponins at lower concentrations than older tests. Careful clinical assessment is therefore all the more crucial.

- Lactate dehydrogenase (LDH):
  - This is non-cardiac specific as levels may be raised in other conditions, e.g. haemolysis.
  - It peaks at 4 days, remaining elevated for 1–2 weeks.
  - Since the advent of troponin tests, it is rarely used.
- Aspartate aminotransferase (AST):
  - This is not specific to myocardial damage, with levels also affected in hepatic disorders, thrombotic conditions and skeletal muscle injury.
  - Peak elevation is at 24 hours post myocardial damage, lasting for 4–6 days.
  - Since the advent of troponin tests, it is rarely used.
- Creatine kinase-myocardium bound (CK-MB):
  - Levels may increase and then fall within 72 hours of myocardial damage.
  - CK-MB generally does not rise until 4 hours post infarction, so is generally not used to make the initial diagnosis of an MI.
  - Since the advent of troponin tests, it is rarely used.

6.2 ELECTROCARDIOGRAPHY

COMPONENTS OF AN ELECTROCARDIOGRAM TRACING

- Standard ECG comprises 12 leads, giving 12 individual tracings. This is achieved by placing six electrodes on the chest and one electrode on each limb.
- Chest leads V1, V2, V3, V4, V5 and V6 all look at the heart in the horizontal plane.
- Leads I, II, III, aVL, aVF and aVR look at the heart in the vertical plane.

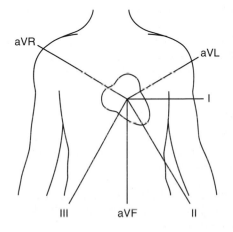

Fig. 6.1 The viewpoint each limb lead has of the heart. Reproduced with permission from Andrew Houghton and David Gray, *Making sense of the ECG, a hands on guide*, 3rd edn. p. 5, Fig. 1.5.

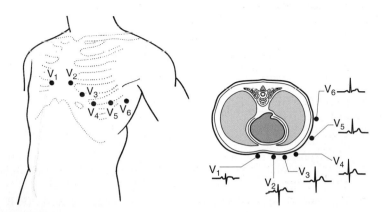

Fig. 6.2 The viewpoint each chest lead has of the heart. Reproduced with permission from Andrew Houghton and David Gray, *Making sense of the ECG, a hands on guide*, 3rd edn. p. 6, Fig. 1.6.

Clinical specialties

- Each ECG electrode picks up the electrical activity of the heart in a particular plane (see Fig. 6.3).
- When electrical activity spreads towards the electrode, the reading will give a positive deflection on the ECG. When the activity spreads away from the electrode, the reading will give a negative deflection on the ECG.
- When combined, these positive and negative deflections depict the cardiac cycle.

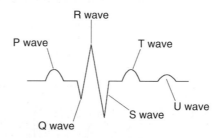

Fig. 6.3 QRS complex. Reproduced with permission from Andrew Houghton and David Gray, *Making sense of the ECG, a hands on guide*, 3rd edn. p. 2, Fig. 1.2.

- It is possible to identify the territory of an acute myocardial infarction by assessing which leads show changes:

Table 6.2 Cardiac territories by ECG leads.

LEADS	TERRITORY THE LEAD REPRESENTS
V1, V2, V3, V4	Right ventricle and septum (anterior surface of heart) – mostly supplied by the left anterior descending artery (LAD)
V5, V6, aVL, I	Left ventricle (lateral surface of the heart) – mostly supplied by the left circumflex artery (LCx)
II, III, aVF	Inferior surface of the heart – mostly supplied by the right coronary artery (RCA)
aVR	Right atrium

CALCULATING THE RATE FROM AN ECG

- One large square of the ECG recording paper is equivalent to 0.2 seconds.
  - ECG recording normally runs at a rate of 25 mm/second.
  - This equates to five large squares per second and 300 per minute.
- Hence, when running at 25 mm/second, the ventricular heart rate can be calculated by either:
  - counting the number of large squares between two R waves (R-R interval), and dividing 300 by this number:
    - e.g. if the R-R interval is two large squares, the heart rate would be 300/2 = 150 beats/min;

- counting the number of small squares between two R waves, and dividing 1500 by this number:
  - e.g. if the R-R interval is 10 small squares, the heart rate would be 1500/10 = 150 beats/min.
- Tachycardia = heart rate > 100 beats/min.
- Bradycardia = heart rate < 60 beats/min (or < 50 beats/min during sleep).

MICRO-facts

With irregular heart rhythms, to calculate the heart rate, work out the average number of squares between several R-R intervals, and use this in your calculation of the heart rate.

ASSESSING THE RHYTHM FROM AN ECG

- This is assessed by viewing P waves and their relationship to the QRS complex.
- Sinus rhythm:
  - The rhythm originates in the sinus node and conducts to the ventricles.
  - The cardinal features of sinus rhythm include:
    - P wave shows positive deflection in leads I and II;
    - each P wave followed by a QRS complex, with a normal fixed interval in between;
    - normal heart rate is 60–99 beats/min.
- Sinus arrhythmia:
  - Describes a sinus rhythm with the variation of heart rate that occurs during inspiration and expiration.
  - There is beat-to-beat variation in the R-R interval, with the rate normally increasing in inspiration, due to the vagal response to increased venous return to the heart.
- Sinus tachycardia:
  - Describes a sinus rhythm with a heart rate > 100 beats/min.
- Sinus bradycardia:
  - Describes a sinus rhythm with a heart rate < 60 beats/min.
- Atrial fibrillation:
  - The most commonly sustained rhythm disorder characterized by uncoordinated atrial activity.
    - ECG findings:
      - P waves absent, ± oscillating baseline fibrillating (f) waves;
      - atrial rate 350–600 beats/min;
      - irregular ventricular rhythm.

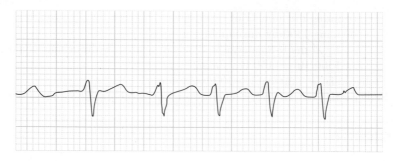

Fig. 6.4 Atrial fibrillation.

- Atrial flutter:
    - This is due to a re-entrant circuit in the right atrium with secondary activation of the left atrium.
    - ECG findings:
        - undulating, 'saw-toothed' baseline flutter (F) waves;
        - atrial rate of almost exactly 300 beats/min;
        - usually regular ventricular rhythm with varying degrees of non-conductance through the AV node:
            - 2:1 block would give rate of 150 beats/min, 4:1 block would give rate of 75 beats/min.

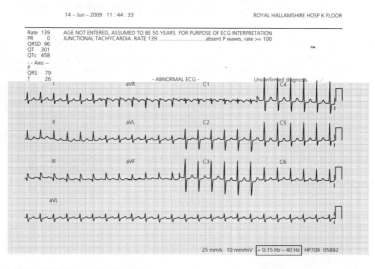

Fig. 6.5 Atrial flutter with 2:1 block.

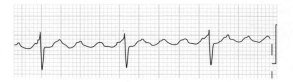

Fig. 6.6 Atrial flutter waves with 3:1 block and flutter waves visible.

- Heart block:
  - First-degree heart block:
    - each QRS complex is preceded by a P wave;
    - the PR interval is prolonged >0.2 s (five small squares), yet remains constant.
  - Second-degree heart block (three main types)
    - Mobitz type I (Wenckebach phenomenon):
      ○ initial PR interval is normal, but progressively lengthens with each successive beat, until eventually there is a dropped beat and a QRS complex does not follow a P wave;
      ○ PR interval then returns to normal and the cycle repeats itself.
    - Mobitz type II.
      ○ intermittent failure of conduction of a P wave;
      ○ PR interval is constant but may be prolonged or normal;
      ○ intermittent conduction of a P wave, so periodically a P wave will not be followed by a QRS complex.
    - Fixed degree of atrioventricular block:
      ○ QRS complex is only seen after a set number of P waves, e.g. in 3:1 block, a QRS complex occurs after every third P wave (three P waves for every QRS complex).
    - Third-degree heart block:
      ○ complete failure of conduction between sino-atrial (SA) node and atrioventricular (AV) node;
      ○ P wave and QRS rates are regular, but unrelated;
      ○ P wave rate may be normal, e.g. 75 per minute;
      ○ QRS rate is often around 35 beats/min, with wide QRS complexes indicating the slow intrinsic ventricular rate.

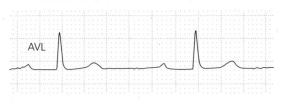

Fig. 6.7 First-degree heart block with bradycardia.

Clinical specialties

Table 6.3 Calculating the axis on the ECG.

LEADS	NORMAL	RIGHT AXIS DEVIATION	LEFT AXIS DEVIATION
I	Positive	Negative	Positive
II	Positive	Positive or negative	Negative
III	Positive or negative	Positive	Negative

ASSESSING THE CARDIAC AXIS FROM AN ECG

- Cardiac axis refers to the mean direction of the wave of ventricular depolarization in the vertical plane.
- It may be normal, deviated to the right or deviated to the left.
- The simplest method of calculating the cardiac axis is to review leads I, II and III.

ASSESSING THE BASIC COMPONENTS OF AN ECG CARDIAC WAVE

P wave

- Represents atrial depolarization.
- Characteristics:
  - Amplitude rarely exceeds two and a half small squares (0.25 mV).
  - Duration should not exceed three small squares (0.12 seconds).
  - Positive/upright in leads I and II, and inverted in aVR.
  - Sinus P waves best viewed in leads II and V1.
  - Often biphasic in lead V1-positive deflection of right atrial depolarization and negative with the left atrial depolarization.
- Pathology:
  - P-mitrale
    - Wide P wave with a pronounced notch (bifid P wave).
    - Usually pathological—seen in association with left atrial enlargement (e.g. mitral stenosis).
  - P-pulmonale
    - Tall, peaked P waves (height > 2.5 mm) in leads II, III and aVF.
    - Occurs transiently in right atrial enlargement (e.g. tricuspid stenosis, pulmonary hypertension) or with pulmonary embolism.

MICRO-facts

A negative P wave in lead I may be due to, in order of likelihood:
1. incorrect lead positions (left and right arm leads being swapped);
2. dextrocardia;
3. abnormal atrial rhythms.

PR interval

- Represents time conduction of electrical signal through the atrioventricular node (AVN), bundle of His, bundle branches and Purkinje fibres.
  - Characteristics:
    - Measured from the beginning of the P wave to the first deflection of QRS complex.
    - Normal duration is three to five small squares (0.12–0.20 seconds).
  - Pathology:
    - Abnormalities in the conducting system may prolong the PR interval due to transmission delays (e.g. heart block).
    - Wolff–Parkinson–White syndrome has a shortened PR interval with a slurred upstroke to the R wave (known as a delta wave). This is due to an accessory pathway, the bundle of Kent, linking the atrium and ventricle.

QRS complex

- Represents ventricular depolarization.
- Normal duration is less than three small squares (<0.12 seconds), measured in the lead with the widest complex.
- Wide QRS complexes (>0.12 seconds) indicate abnormal conduction through ventricles (e.g. bundle branch blocks).
- Single broad QRS complexes in the context of an otherwise normal ECG are usually ventricular ectopic beats, which have no clinical significance in themselves.
- Increase in QRS height may be caused by an increase of left or right ventricular muscle mass.

MICRO-facts

Note the following nomenclature of the QRS complex:

- Q wave is any initial negative deflection
- R wave is any positive deflection
- S wave is any negative deflection after the R wave

Table 6.4 Features of left and right bundle branch block (BBB).

RBBB	LBBB
QRS >0.2 s in duration	QRS >0.2 s in duration
Secondary R wave (two upward deflections = RSR pattern) in V1 or V2	Broad monophasic R wave in leads I, V5 and V6
Wide slurred S wave in leads I, V5 and V6	Absent Q waves in leads V5 and V6

MICRO-facts

In bundle branch block, remember the term 'WiLLiaM MaRRoW'

- **WiLLiaM** – in LBBB, the QRS is **W** shaped in V1 and **M** shaped in V6.
- **MaRRoW**– in RBBB, the QRS is **M** shaped in V1 and **W** shaped in V6.

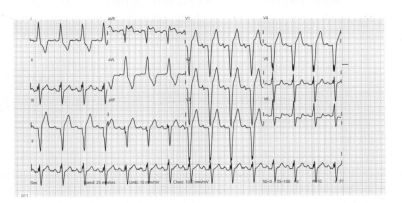

Fig. 6.8 Left bundle branch block. Note this ECG also shows first-degree heart block.

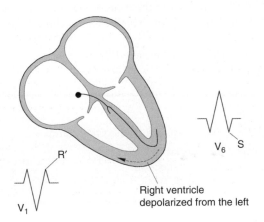

Fig. 6.9 Right bundle branch block. Reproduced with permission from Andrew Houghton and David Gray, *Making sense of the ECG, a hands on guide*, 3rd edn. p. 151, Fig. 8.14.

> **MICRO-print**
> **Cornell criteria for LVH**
> Sum of S wave depth in V3 and R wave height in aVL.
> Diagnostic values are:
> - Men: >28 mm
> - Women: >20 mm

- Right ventricular hypertrophy:
    - This is best seen in the right ventricular lead (V1).
    - R wave height exceeds depth of Q or S wave (QRS complex becomes positive in V1) – always abnormal.
    - Deep S wave in V6. Can be associated with right axis deviation and peaked P waves.
- Left ventricular hypertrophy:
    - Tall R waves in V5 and V6 and deep S wave in V1 or V2.
    - Inverted T waves in lateral leads.
    - Sometimes associated with left axis deviation.
- Pathological Q waves:
    - >0.04 s (one small square) in width.
    - More than 2 mm (2 small squares) deep.
    - Indicates previous myocardial infarction.
    - The pathological Q wave lead indicates the location of affected myocardium (see earlier Table 6.2).
    - Presence of Q waves does not indicate the age of the infarct; once developed, a Q wave persists, although it may change over time.

> **MICRO-facts**
> In LBBB, the only other information that can be obtained from the ECG is the ventricular rate and heart rhythm. Do not attempt to comment on anything else, including ST segments.

ST segment
- Represents the period between the end of ventricular depolarization and beginning of ventricular repolarization.
- Characteristics:
    - ST segment lies between end of the QRS complex and beginning of the T wave.
    - Isoelectric – should be level with the 'TP segment'.

Clinical specialties

- Normally horizontal, although it may slope upwards slightly to merge with the T wave = high take off.
- Should measure 80 ms (2 mm) after the J point.
- Non-pathological elevation of the ST segment is also associated with benign early repolarization, particularly common in men, athletes and Afro-Caribbeans.

MICRO-facts

Changes in STEMI

- A subtle increase in T-wave amplitude – **hyperacute T waves.**
- **ST segment elevation** follows and is the most obvious change.
- Subsequently, **pathological Q waves** appear and the **T wave becomes inverted**.
- The ST segment then returns to baseline.
  - The whole process takes from 24-48 hours.
  - Infarction may abort if a thrombus is cleared spontaneously, in which case pathological Q waves may not form: an 'aborted STEMI' or subendocardial infarction.
  - The aim of primary percutaneous coronary intervention (PCI) is to prevent full-thickness myocardial damage (as indicated by pathological Q waves) by reopening an occluded coronary artery.
  - Prompt PCI may return the ECG to normal.

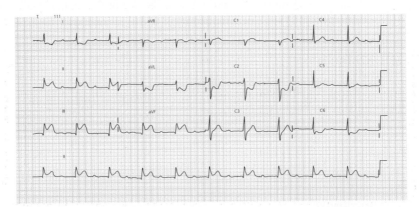

Fig. 6.10 Inferior ST segment elevation myocardial infarction with ST elevation in leads II, III and AVF and reciprocal ST depression in leads I, AVL, V2 and V6. This image is provided courtesy of Sheffield Teaching Hospitals Foundation Trust.

- Pathology:
  - **Elevated** ST segment
    - Indicates acute myocardial injury e.g. acute myocardial infarction or myopericarditis.
    - ST segment elevation in particular leads indicates the region of myocardium that is damaged (see Table 6.2).
    - Persistent ST elevation after 1 week indicates either re-infarction, or ventricular aneurysm.
    - Myopericarditis is not localized and hence causes widespread ST elevation, usually with a concave or 'saddle-shaped' profile compared with convex ST elevation seen in STEMI.

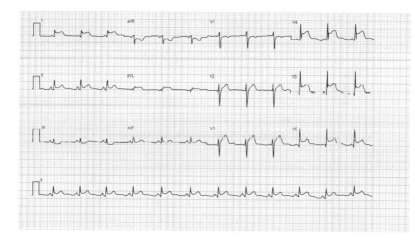

Fig. 6.11 Myopericarditis with widespread concave ST elevation.

MICRO-print

Pericarditis is often mentioned as the cause of ECG appearances such as in Fig. 6.11. The pericardium however has no contractile cells, and therefore produces no ECG changes by itself. **Myocarditis**, which often occurs with pericarditis (myopericarditis), is the cause of the ECG changes, and may also lead to a troponin rise. This ECG is often confused with an acute coronary syndrome, but the widespread concave ST elevation with no reciprocal ST depression gives the diagnosis.

- **Depressed** ST segment
  - Usually associated with upright T wave, is a sign of myocardial ischaemia
  - May appear on an exercise ECG, indicating ischaemia.

Clinical specialties

- Ventricular hypertrophy may lead to a 'strain' pattern of ST depression on the ECG.
- In acute ST elevation myocardial infarction, reciprocal ST depression may be present in leads opposite to those with ST elevation.
- Digoxin toxicity is characterized by 'reverse tick' ST segment depression.
- Posterior ST elevation myocardial infarction causes ST depression in leads V1–3. This is in fact reciprocal ST depression; if posterior chest leads are used (V7–9) ST elevation is seen.

T wave

- Represents ventricular repolarization.
- Characteristics:
  - Normally asymmetrical, with the first half sloping more than the second half.
  - T-wave orientation usually inverted in leads aVR and V1.
  - V2 may be inverted in the young.
  - V3 may be inverted in Afro-Caribbeans.
  - No widely accepted criteria exist regarding T-wave amplitude, but, as a general rule, should be less than two-thirds of the height of the neighbouring R wave.
- Pathology:
  - Inversion of T waves
    - May be normal in particular leads (see earlier under Characteristics).
    - May indicate ischaemia from a previous myocardial infarction, whereby the T-wave inversion is a permanent change on the ECG.
    - May indicate acute ischaemia during a non-ST elevation myocardial infarction (NSTEMI) or positive exercise test.
    - May occur in ventricular hypertrophy, with T-wave inversion in leads V5, V6, II and aVL in left ventricular hypertrophy, and leads V1, V2 and V3 in right ventricular hypertrophy.
    - The abnormal path of depolarization of bundle branch block is usually associated with abnormal repolarization, and hence inverted T waves may be associated, and have no significance in themselves.
    - Digoxin may cause T-wave inversion. When starting digoxin therapy, it is useful to perform an ECG to prevent future confusion of T-wave inversion.
  - Potassium abnormalities
    - Hyperkalaemia; tall, tented P waves.
    - Hypokalaemia; flat, broad T waves.

QT interval
- Represents the total time of ventricular depolarization and repolarization.
- Characteristics:
  - Measured from beginning of QRS interval to end of T wave, best measured in lead aVL to prevent confusion with any prominent U waves.
  - Between 0.35 and 0.45 seconds.
  - Should not be more than half of the interval between adjacent R waves (R-R interval).
  - Increases slightly with age and tends to be longer in women.
- Pathology:
  - The QT interval may be prolonged due to serum chemical imbalances, e.g. hypokalaemia, hypocalcaemia.
  - Drug therapies, including amiodarone, tricyclic antidepressants, quinidine, quinine, flecainide and sotalol, may prolong the QT interval.
  - Long QT syndrome is a channelopathy, where the QTc value is >450 ms.

Table 6.5 ECG changes found with potassium abnormalities.

HYPERKALAEMIA	HYPOKALAEMIA
Tall, tented T waves	Flat, broad T waves
Loss of P waves	ST depression
Broad QRS complex	Long QT interval
Sine-wave shaped ECG	Ventricular dysrhythmias
Cardiac arrest rhythms	

MICRO-print
QT interval lengthens as the heart rate slows. Thus when measuring QT intervals, the rate must be taken into account. QTc is the corrected QT interval for heart rate: Bazett's formula.

U waves
- These represent repolarization of the mid-myocardial cells and the His–Purkinje system.
- Characteristics:
  - Small deflection following the T wave. Generally positive deflection apart from in aVR, and most prominent in V2–V4.
  - Many ECGs do not have U waves.
  - May be normal in athletes.
  - Associated with hypercalcaemia and hypokalaemia.

Clinical specialties

MICRO-facts

Have an orderly system when interpreting and presenting ECGs, e.g.

- Patient details (name, age, date of birth, sex)
- ECG details (date/time taken, reason for ECG and type of ECG)
- Heart rate
- Heart rhythm
- Cardiac axis
- Components of the ECG complex in order – P, PR, QRS, ST, T, QT
- Summary of your findings.

CARDIAC ARREST RHYTHMS

Needless to say, these are medical emergencies and basic and advanced life support should be commenced immediately in any arrest situation.

MICRO-reference

European Resuscitation Council. **Guidelines for Resuscitation**. 2010. http://www.cprguidelines.eu/2010/ (accessed 23/08/2011).

- Ventricular fibrillation (VF):
  - A common initial arrhythmia in cardiac arrest.
  - Uncoordinated ventricular activity leads to loss of cardiac output and circulatory arrest.
  - This rhythm is shockable and therefore prompt defibrillation is essential to attempt to cardiovert the heart back to sinus rhythm.
  - Prolonged VF may change to a non-shockable rhythm with time, and these carry a much worse prognosis. Early defibrillation therefore is a priority.

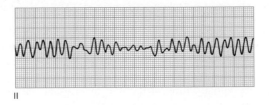

II

Fig. 6.12 Ventricular fibrillation. Reproduced with permission from Andrew Houghton and David Gray, *Making sense of the ECG, a hands on guide*, 3rd edn. p. 259, Fig. 17.2.

- Pulseless ventricular tachycardia (VT):
  - The first word here is key – 'pulseless'; it is possible to have VT without cardiac arrest, and therefore as with any emergency situation

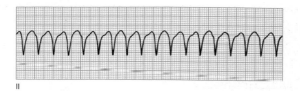

Fig. 6.13 Ventricular tachycardia. Reproduced with permission from Andrew Houghton and David Gray, *Making sense of the ECG, a hands on guide*, 3rd edn, page 259, Fig. 17.3.

careful Airway, Breathing, Circulation, Disability, Exposure (ABCDE) assessment is essential.
- VT is a broad complex tachycardia, i.e. QRS width >3 small squares.
- There are two key types of ventricular tachycardia:
  - **monomorphic,** which has a single constant QRS morphology (see Fig. 6.13);
  - **polymorphic,** also known as torsades de pointes, which has a variable QRS morphology (see Fig. 6.14).
- **Pulseless VT** is a shockable rhythm and urgent defibrillation is a priority.

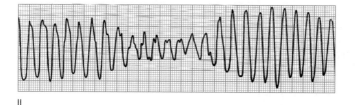

Fig. 6.14 Torsades de pointes. Reproduced with permission from Andrew Houghton and David Gray, *Making sense of the ECG, a hands on guide*, 3rd edn. p. 56, Fig. 3.20

- Asystole:
  - No significant electrical activity is present, although there is a fluctuating baseline.
  - If there is simply a 'flat line' then it is highly likely that an ECG lead has become unattached!
  - This is a non-shockable rhythm and therefore adrenaline is the first-line Advanced drug along with highquality -Basic Life Support, i.e. CPR.
- Pulseless electrical activity (PEA):
  - Once again, ABC assessment is essential to diagnose this arrhythmia.
  - **Any** ECG trace other than those mentioned above may be present, from sinus rhythm to left bundle branch block.
  - This is sometimes known as electromechanical dissociation, with no cardiac muscle activity or output but a seemingly normal ECG.
  - Clinical assessment of the patient is key!

Clinical specialties

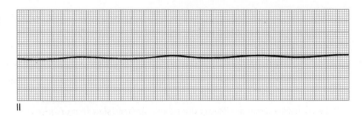

II

Fig. 6.15 Asystole. Reproduced with permission from Andrew Houghton and David Gray, *Making sense of the ECG, a hands on guide*, 3rd edn. p. 261, Fig. 17.4.

6.3 OTHER COMMON CARDIOLOGY INVESTIGATIONS

CARDIAC RADIOLOGY

This section will aim to cover a brief overview of cardiospecific radiology; however, for more in-depth information, please refer to Chapter 5, Radiology.

- Cardiac failure:
  - Plain chest radiograph (remember ABCDE mnemonic):
    - A for alveolar bat's wings
    - B for Kerley B lines (horizontal lines of fluid-filled septae at the costophrenic angles)
    - C for cardiomegaly (indicating enlarged left ventricle)
    - D for upper lobe diversion (arteriolar vasoconstriction due to alveolar hypoxia)
    - E for pleural effusions.
- Pericardial effusion:
  - Plain chest radiograph
    - illustrates symmetrically enlarged and globular cardiac shadow with significant effusion (> 250 mL);
    - should be suspected when there is a rapid serial increase in the cardiac shadow with normal pulmonary vasculature.
  - Echocardiography
    - gold standard for diagnosing pericardial effusions;
    - effusion visible as echo-free areas surrounding heart.
  - CT
    - may contribute to identifying the underlying cause of the effusion.
  - MRI
    - accurate in diagnosing pericardial effusion, with additional imaging of cardiothoracic area.
- Deep vein thrombosis:
  - Colour Doppler ultrasound

- thrombus may be seen within vessel lumen, often accompanied by reduced or absent blood flow.
  - Venography
    - contrast administered to patient's foot vein with a tourniquet placed at the ankle and above the knee to force the contrast into the deep veins. Now virtually never performed;
    - a filling defect is then seen when a thrombus is present.
- Abdominal aortic aneurysm (AAA):
  - Plain abdominal radiograph
    - calcification of the abdominal aorta.
  - Ultrasound
    - used in diagnosis and monitoring of AAA;
    - >5.5 cm diameter leads to an increased risk of rupture.
  - CT/MRI
    - ideal for pre-operative assessment to evaluate the exact anatomical approach to take along with assessment of renal artery involvement.
- Aortic thoracic dissection:
  - Plain chest radiograph
    - shows a widened mediastinum or pleural cap, suggesting aortic dissection.
  - CT/MRI
    - needed to confirm and diagnose dissection. This is usually done by a CT scan, rarely by an MRI.
- Cardiac calcification:
  - Plain chest radiographs
    - indicated on radiographs by increased 'whiteness';
    - pericardial calcification seen as a 'whitening' of the border of the heart in a curvilinear fashion;
    - myocardial calcification typically seen at apex of heart;
    - valve calcification only seen with extensive calcification, indicating stenosis of the valve. Aortic and mitral valves most commonly affected.

EXERCISE ELECTROCARDIOGRAPHY

- Indications:
  - After MI to evaluate prognosis and/or aid rehabilitation.
  - Pre- and post-revascularization.
  - Evaluation of arrhythmias.
  - Diagnosis of ischemic heart disease with atypical chest pain symptoms.
- Contraindications:
  - ECG not interpretable
    - LBBB;
    - LVH with strain;
    - digoxin;
    - right ventricular pacemaker.

Clinical specialties

- Patient unable to exercise;
    - immobility, e.g. severe osteoarthritis;
    - aortic stenosis;
    - hypertrophic obstructive cardiomyopathy (HOCM) – it is dangerous to exercise;
    - left ventricular failure;
    - severe hypertension;
    - aortic dissection;
    - recent acute coronary syndrome;
    - peripheral vascular disease;
    - second- or third-degree heart block.
- Patient preparation:
    - All patients must be seen and examined prior to the exercise test to ensure no contraindications.
    - Explain the test and its risks to the patient to obtain consent. Mortality risk is approximately 0.5–1/10 000.
    - Some antihypertensives and antianginal medications are stopped prior to the test, e.g. beta-blockers.
    - Resuscitation equipment should always be available throughout the procedure.
- Procedure outline:
    - Aim of exercise test is to stress the cardiovascular system.
    - If sufficient blood is not supplied to the myocardium under stress, the tissue becomes ischaemic and the ECG will change.
    - The best method of exercise is a treadmill test.
    - The Bruce protocol is often employed giving incrementally higher speeds and gradients up to 9 minutes in total.
    - In patients unable to exercise, pharmacological agents (adenosine or dobutamine) may be used to increase heart rate and stress the heart.
    - 12-lead ECG, blood pressure and heart rate are measured before, during and after the test until they return to pre-exercise levels.
- Reasons for terminating the test:
    - Attainment of maximal heart rate (220 beats/min – patient's age).
    - Completion of all stages of test with no symptoms without reaching maximal heart rate.
    - Chest pain, excessive fatigue or shortness of breath, dizziness, syncope, arrhythmias.
    - ST segment depression (> 1.5 mm) or elevation at 2 mm after the J point.
    - ST segment elevation.
- Indicators of a positive result:
    - ST segment depression > 1.5 mm at 2 mm after the J point.
    - ST segment elevation.
    - Classical angina pectoris.

- Arrhythmias.
- Fall in blood pressure of more than 15 mmHg, or failure to rise.

ECHOCARDIOGRAPHY

- Transthoracic echocardiography (TTE):
  - Views the heart in two dimensions and three dimensions, and with Doppler effects.
  - Useful for assessing:
    - valve structure and function;
    - atrial/ventricular sizes and function (e.g. wall thickness and contractility);
    - congenital cardiac malformations;
    - pericardial disease;
    - pulmonary hypertension (estimated pulmonary artery pressure);
  - Less accurate for viewing posterior cardiac structures, e.g. the mitral valve, as these are further from the transducer.
  - Advantage over TOE is its relative simplicity (non-invasive) and the reduced procedure time.
- Transoesophageal echocardiography (TOE):
  - TOE uses a flexible endoscope with a two-dimensional transducer at the tip, introduced into the oesophagus and stomach.
  - This gives clearer images than TTE due to the proximity to the heart.
  - Indications for TOE:
    - intracardiac thrombus and cardiac masses;
    - pericardial disease and masses;
    - aortic pathology;
    - valve defects/disease (vegetations, regurgitation, stenosis);
    - congenital heart lesions;
    - during cardiac surgery to give information on valve function and ventricular function;
    - poor TTE views.
  - TOE procedure/preparation:
    - local anaesthesia, with additional IV sedation if required;
    - the patients will have fasted 6 hours prior to the procedure;
    - oxygen and wall suction should always be available;
    - mouth guard to protect the teeth;
    - ECG monitoring for assessment of images with the cardiac cycle.
  - Complications are rare ($<0.01\%$), but may include:
    - oesophageal rupture;
    - laryngospasm;
    - ventricular arrhythmias;
    - severe hypoxia.

Clinical specialties

NUCLEAR IMAGING

- Concept:
    - Looks at the uptake of isotopes by the cardiac muscle, and in doing so assesses myocardial contractility and oxygen supply.
    - A quantitative estimate of ventricular function (expressed as ejection fraction) and reversibility of ischaemia are also detectable.
- Indications:
    - If exercise ECG is equivocal and confirmation of reversible ischaemia is required prior to angiography.
    - If patient cannot perform exercise ECG test due to poor mobility.
    - In all other cases, exercise ECG testing is the first-line investigation.
- Benefits:
    - Non-invasive.
    - More sensitive than exercise testing alone.
- Disadvantages:
    - Expensive.
    - Requires radiation exposure.
    - Lengthy procedure (1- or 2-day protocol).
    - May give false positive result in diffuse ischaemic disease.

MICRO-print

- MUGA (multigated acquisition) scans are nuclear imaging scans that concentrate on imaging the cardiac blood pool alongside an ECG to correlate the different stages of the cardiac cycle, and ultimately assess cardiac function.
- PET (positron emission tomography) scans may be used when other conventional nuclear imaging and angiography techniques prove to be equivocal.

CARDIAC CATHETERIZATION ANGIOGRAMS AND ANGIOPLASTY

- Indications:
    - Suspected acute STEMI – primary percutaneous coronary intervention (PCI).
    - Recent NSTEMI – usually within 48 hours.
    - Positive exercise test or myocardial imaging scan.
    - Recent cardiac arrest.
    - Pre-operatively prior to coronary artery bypass surgery.
    - Annual review after cardiac transplantation.
    - Occupational reasons (e.g. airline pilots).
    - High-risk, symptomatic patients with ischaemic heart disease.
    - Assessment of pulmonary hypertension (right heart catheter).

- Technique:
    - Access to right heart gained via femoral, subclavian or internal jugular veins.
    - Access to left heart gained via femoral, brachial or radial artery.
    - Catheters passed through vessels to desired location via fluoroscopic X-ray guidance.
    - Pressure of chambers or vessels may be recorded.
    - Oxygen saturation of blood at particular locations can be measured.
    - Patency of arteries (coronary angiography) may be assessed with radio-opaque contrast.
    - Balloon angioplasty with or without stenting may be performed to open up stenoses in coronary arteries.
    - Contractility of ventricles and aortic root anatomy can be assessed using radio-opaque contrast.
    - Cardiac biopsies may also be taken.
- Potential risks:
    - Haemorrhage from puncture site.
    - Formation of pseudoaneurysm.
    - Infection of puncture site or rarely septicaemia.
    - Allergic reaction to contrast.
    - Arrhythmias.
    - Thrombosis of artery.
    - Pericardial tamponade if vessel dissection or myocardial tear.
    - Displacement of atherosclerotic fragments leading to MI, cerebro-vascular event, etc.
- Results:
    - Images are recorded using videofluoroscopy recording or cine camera.

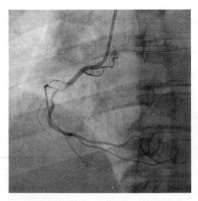

Fig. 6.16 Right coronary angiogram showing significant mid vessel stenosis. Courtesy of Dr Ian Hall, Consultant Cardiologist, Northern General Hospital, Sheffield.

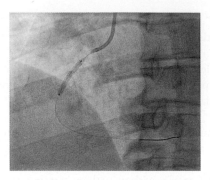

Fig. 6.17 Right coronary angiogram showing stent inflation with angioplasty balloon. Courtesy of Dr Ian Hall, Consultant Cardiologist, Northern General Hospital, Sheffield.

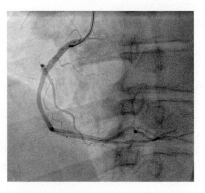

Fig. 6.18 Right coronary angiogram showing the final result of angioplasty with excellent right coronary flow and no residual mid vessel stenosis. Courtesy of Dr Ian Hall, Consultant Cardiologist, Northern General Hospital, Sheffield.

MICRO-print

Other specialized investigations employed in cardiology include:

- **Tilt-table testing**: aids diagnosis of patients experiencing syncope. The aim is to reproduce the syncopal event while the patient is connected to BP and ECG monitors.
- **Cardiac magnetic resonance imaging**: non-invasive test that can view each stage of the cardiac cycle with reference to the patient's ECG trace. It is used to investigate ischaemic and structural heart disease.
- **Computed tomography**: this is used along with MRI because of their high sensitivity for excluding aortic dissections. CT angiography is also increasingly employed to view the coronary vessels, but patients must be beta-blocked prior to this procedure, with a heart rate < 64 beats/minute.

MICRO-case

Interpret the ECG in Fig 6.19 from a 70-year-old man with a history of smoking and hypertension. He is currently asymptomatic, and this trace was taken at a pre-operative assessment clinic for a routine cholecystectomy.

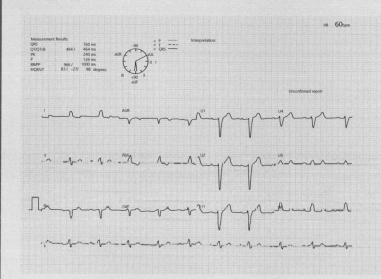

Fig. 6.19

- Demographic details
  - Male, Chester Payne, DOB 29/10/1940, Hospital number XX4571
  - Smoker, hypertension
- ECG details: Routine pre-op ECG for cholecystectomy
- Heart Rate: 60 beats/min
- Rhythm: Sinus rhythm
- Axis: Normal
- Components of the ECG:
  - P waves are normal;
  - PR interval is **prolonged** at six small squares;
  - QRS complex is **broad** at four small squares, **left bundle branch block** present;
  - Therefore, we cannot comment on ST segment or T waves.
- Summary
  - A routine pre-operative ECG in a smoker with hypertension showing sinus rhythm at 60 beats/min with first-degree heart block and left bundle branch block.

continued...

Clinical specialties

continued...

Learning points

- Many patients with abnormal ECGs will be asymptomatic.
- There may be more than one abnormality on an ECG.
- A systematic approach is essential so as not to miss any pathology.
- Left bundle branch block is almost invariably associated with underlying pathology, and therefore this patient should have further assessment prior to his operation.

MICRO-reference

National Institute of Clinical Excellence. Chronic heart failure: National Guidelines for diagnosis and management in primary and secondary care. http://guidance.nice.org.uk/CG108/Guidance/pdf/English (accessed 23/08/2011).

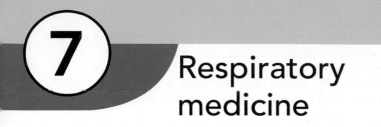

Respiratory medicine

7.1 ARTERIAL BLOOD GAS ANALYSIS

> ### MICRO-facts
>
> Arterial blood gas sampling is painful. Much of the information given by the test may be gleaned through other methods: a venous sample may demonstrate acidosis with low bicarbonate, e.g. in DKA, and pulse oximetry gives a reliable indication of oxygenation. Before attempting the procedure, think whether the information you are looking for could be found with another test.

ARTERIAL BLOOD GAS SAMPLING

- Indications:
  - Dyspnoea/tachypnea.
  - Low blood oxygen saturations (SaO_2).
  - Suspected respiratory or metabolic abnormality.
- Contraindications:
  - For radial puncture
    - poor ulnar circulation;
    - previous arterial harvesting, e.g. for coronary artery bypass grafting (CABG).
- Sites for sampling:
  - Radial is preferred site, although ulnar, brachial or femoral arteries may be used.
  - Patients on high-dependency unit or intensive treatment unit often have long-term arterial lines *in situ*, from which arterial blood may be taken.
- Preparations:
  - Perform Allen's test to assess collateral circulation to hand.
  - Clean puncture site with alcohol swab.
  - Apply pressure to site for 5 minutes following procedure.

- Complications:
    - Haematoma at puncture site, ischaemia to hand if poor collateral circulation (0.09%), bleeding, infection.
- Analysis time:
    - Modern ABG analysers can give results in $\sim$ 1 minute.
    - Time taken for doctor to reach machine is variable!

MICRO-facts

Normal values for an ABG

- pH   7.35–7.45
- PaO_2 11–13 kPa
- $PaCO_2$ 4.7–6.0 kPa
- HCO_3^- 22–28 mmol/L
- Base excess   −2 to +2 mmol/L
- Anion gap   12–16 mmol/L

---

pH ANALYSIS

- Low blood pH is termed acidaemia.
- High blood pH is termed an alkalaemia.
- CO_2 makes blood acidic, becoming carbonic acid when dissolved.
- HCO_3^- makes blood alkaline, buffering free H^+ ions.
- Disorders of pH balance are classified into four main types:
    1) respiratory acidosis;
    2) respiratory alkalosis;
    3) metabolic acidosis;
    4) metabolic alkalosis.
- In each of the first two disorders, ventilation is either excessive or inadequate, leading to low or high $PaCO_2$ levels.
- In the second two disorders, serum H^+ ion concentration is deranged by:
    - excess acid production or ingestion, e.g. lactic acid in sepsis;
    - acid loss, e.g. in vomiting – classically with pyloric stenosis;
    - bicarbonate loss, e.g. in diarrhoea;
    - poor renal function – either inadequate or excessive bicarbonate loss.
- In respiratory disorders, HCO_3^- concentrations will change as the kidney compensates for the abnormality.
- In metabolic disorders, $PaCO_2$ concentrations will change as ventilation is increased or decreased to compensate for the abnormality.
- Respiratory acidosis arises due to any cause of hypoventilation and therefore CO_2 retention, e.g. pneumonia, opiate overdose, stroke, etc.
- Respiratory alkalosis is due to hyperventilation, e.g. in panic attacks.
- Metabolic alkalosis may be due to:

- gastrointestinal (GI) losses, e.g. vomiting;
- hyperaldosteronism;
- diuretics;
- hypercalcaemia;
- excess bicarbonate ingestion.

Table 7.1 Arterial blood gas analysis.

DISORDER OF pH	pH	$PaCO_2$	HCO_3^-	PRIMARY PROBLEM	COMPENSATION
Respiratory acidosis	↓	↑	↑	↓ Ventilation	Renal
Respiratory alkalosis	↑	↓	↓	↑ Ventilation	Renal
Metabolic acidosis	↓	↓	↓	E g sepsis DKA	↑ Ventilation, renal
Metabolic alkalosis	↑	↔/↑	↑	E.g. vomiting	↓ Ventilation, renal

DKA, diabetic ketoacidosis.

- Metabolic acidosis has many causes that may be differentiated by calculating the **anion gap**.
- This is calculated as follows:

$$(Na^+ + K^+) - (Cl^- + HCO_3^-)$$

- Diseases affecting concentrations of these and other simple ions, e.g. calcium, magnesium and phosphate, lead to an acidosis with a low or normal anion gap.
- A high anion gap is due to the presence of acids which are not routinely measured, e.g. lactate.

Table 7.2 Causes of high and low anion gaps.

NORMAL/LOW ANION GAP	HIGH ANION GAP
Renal tubular acidosis	Ketoacidosis
Loss of HCO_3^-, e.g. in diarrhoea	Lactic acidosis
Excess normal (0.9%) saline	Ingestion of salicylate, methanol, ethylene glycol
Drugs, e.g. acetazolamide	Renal failure

Clinical specialties

PaO_2

- This is important in the assessment of respiratory illness.
- A value of <8 kPa with a normal or low $PaCO_2$ would indicate type I respiratory failure.
- It is used to guide oxygen therapy.
- **It must** be interpreted with reference to inspired FiO_2.
    - With normal lung function, one would expect PaO_2 to be roughly 10 kPa lower than inspired FiO_2, e.g. if FiO_2 40%, PaO_2 should be ~ 30 kPa.
    - Lung pathology will decrease PaO_2, and the difference between the expected and actual values indicates severity of illness.
    - A PaO_2 of 10 kPa on room air (FiO_2 21%) is not worrying, whereas on an FiO_2 of 60% it could precipitate a phone call to the intensive treatment unit!

> **MICRO-reference**
>
> O'Driscoll BR, Howard LS, Davison AG. BTS guideline for emergency oxygen use in adult patients. Thorax 2008; 63 (Suppl 6): vi1–68.

$PaCO_2$

- This is important in assessment of respiratory illness.
- Level of >6.5 kPa in the context of a low PaO_2 indicates type II respiratory failure.
- Low values indicate excessive ventilation, while high levels show inadequate ventilation.

> **MICRO-facts**
>
> **Respiratory failure**
>
> | | PaO_2 | $PaCO_2$ |
> | --- | --- | --- |
> | Type I | <8 kPa ↓ | Normal or ↓ |
> | Type II | <8 kPa ↓ | >6.5 kPa ↑ |

OTHER VALUES

- Lactate, haemoglobin and electrolytes such as Na^+ and K^+ may be measured from venous or arterial samples using some modern blood gas analysers.

- Systems vary and these values may not be as accurate as those from formal laboratory analysis.
- They can, however, give a rapid indication of important abnormalities in the acutely unwell patient.

7.2 PLEURAL FLUID ANALYSIS

PLEURAL ASPIRATION: THORACENTESIS

- Indications:
    - Pleural effusion detected on clinical examination or imaging.
    - Visible on chest radiograph (CXR) if > 200 mL of fluid.
- Contraindications/cautions:
    - Increased risk of bleeding, e.g. haemophilia, deranged clotting function, low platelets.
- Preparations:
    - Full blood count, clotting screen.
    - Sterilization of target area.
    - Imaging – CXR, then either CT or ultrasound scan for localization of effusion.
- Technique:
    - A 21G needle is attached to a syringe and inserted between an intercostal space overlying the effusion, avoiding the neurovascular bundle at the superior border. Now usually performed under ultrasound guidance.
- Complications:
    - Bleeding, infection, damage to intrathoracic organs/nerves, pneumothorax.

TYPES OF FLUID

- The commonest is a simple effusion.
- Blood in pleural space is a haemothorax.
- Lymph in pleural space is a chylothorax.
- Pus in pleural space is an empyema.

PARAMETERS ASSESSED

- Appearance:
    - Straw – normal.
    - Yellow – infection, i.e. parapneumonic effusion.
    - Pus – empyema.
    - Milky – chylothorax.
    - Bloody:

- blood stained – traumatic sample, cancer, pulmonary embolism;
- frank blood – haemothorax, e.g. due to trauma.
- **Odour** – if putrid, consider anaerobic infection.
- Biochemical tests:
  - Protein differentiates transudate from exudate.
  - pH <7.2 indicates empyema.
  - Lactate dehydrogenase differentiates transudate from exudate.
  - Amylase – raised in pancreatitis, may be higher than serum level.
  - Glucose – low in infection, rheumatoid disease and in some malignant effusions.
- Cell count:
  - ↑ White cell count (WCC) $>1000/\mu l$ suggests exudate.
  - ↑ Lymphocytes suggests TB.
  - ↑ Red cell count in malignancy, trauma, haemothorax, PE.
- Microscopy, culture and sensitivity, for bacteria.
- **TB**: auramine phenol or Ziehl–Neelsen stain and mycobacterial culture:
  - Microscopy yield only 10–20%, culture yield only $\sim 40\%$ from pleural fluid therefore sputum or pleural biopsy preferable.
- **Cytology** for investigation of malignancy.
- **Immunology:** anti-nuclear antibody (ANA), complement, rheumatoid factor – not often used as serum levels more reliable.

CAUSES OF A PLEURAL EFFUSION

- History and examination findings are important.
  - Any results should be interpreted in the clinical context.
- Causes of a pleural effusion are divided into two groups:
  - exudates;
  - transudates.
- Determined by Light's criteria for an exudate (98% sensitivity, 83% specificity).
- For simplicity, fluid protein levels are often used in isolation, but this assumes a normal blood protein level (sensitivity 84%, specificity 82.1%).
  - Fluid protein $>30\,g/L$ indicates exudate.
  - Fluid protein $<30\,g/L$ indicates transudate.
- Other indicators are:
  - transudate usually bilateral, exudate usually unilateral;
  - ↑ WCC indicates exudate.
- If the cause is still unclear after standard tests, thoracoscopy and pleural biopsy may be of benefit, as would investigating for PE.
  - No cause is found for $\sim 15\%$ of exudative effusions even after thoracoscopy and pleural biopsy.

Table 7.3 Differential diagnosis of pleural effusion.

TRANSUDATE	EXUDATE
Heart failure by far the commonest cause	Pneumonia – parapneumonic effusion
Liver failure	Empyema
Renal failure	Malignancy – local or metastatic
Hypoalbuminaemia	Tuberculosis
Hypothyroidism (rare)	Pulmonary embolus
Pulmonary embolus (usually an exudate)	Pancreatitis
Sarcoidosis	Connective tissue disorders
	Drug-induced, e.g. amiodarone
	Chylothorax
	Post-coronary artery bypass surgery

7.3 PULMONARY FUNCTION TESTING

PEAK EXPIRATORY FLOW

- Peak expiratory flow (PEF) is defined as:
  - maximal flow rate of exhalation in L/min.
- Indications for PEF are:
  - asthma
    - monitoring;
    - assessment of response to treatment;
    - assessment of severity in the acute setting.
  - It is NOT indicated for chronic obstructive pulmonary disease (COPD).
- Preparations:
  - Height, age and sex are recorded.
  - Patient sits upright or is standing.
  - Full inspiration.
  - Rest, no cigarettes and no inhalers/nebulizers for 1 hour before test.
- Technique:
  - Forced exhalation as hard and fast as possible.
  - Repeated three times with highest value recorded.
  - Usually done three times daily and recorded on a PEF chart.

Clinical specialties

- Measurement:
  - Pointer moves horizontally along scale to show maximal flow rate in L/minute.
  - Compared with a nomogram based on age, sex and height
    - EU nomogram was published in 1989;
    - does not differentiate different ethnic groups.
- Benefits:
  - Quick, easy, cheap and portable.
  - Patients can perform at home and record in diary
    - useful for assessment of treatment response.
  - Readings at home and at work useful for investigation of occupational asthma.
  - Very useful in acute setting.

MICRO-facts

Asthma is reversible with therapy.
COPD is not reversible.

- Limitations/problems:
  - Variable with patient effort.
  - Not as repeatable as spirometry.
  - Normal result when patient well does not exclude disease.
  - Not accurate for diagnosis of asthma
    - Sensitivity only 19–33% for physician-diagnosed asthma.
- Reversibility: indicates asthma:
  - Assessed before and after inhalation of 400 µg of salbutamol.
  - Or assessed before and after 6–8 weeks twice daily inhalation of 200 µg of beclometasone.
  - Or assessed before and after 14 days of 30 mg of oral prednisolone daily.
  - Defined as an improvement of >60 L/min of best PEF.
- Variability:
  - Indicates asthma
    - **diurnal**: PEF usually worse in the morning;
    - **day to day**: climate/occupational factors.

Table 7.4 Comparison of peak expiratory flow (PEF) and spirometry.

PEF	SPIROMETRY
Cheap, widely available, portable	Cheap, widely available
Reversibility: >60 L/min improvement	Reversibility: >400 mL improvement in FEV_1
Normal ranges outdated, not validated for ethnic variation	Normal ranges reliable
Effort dependent	Effort independent
Variable accuracy if repeated	Accurate if repeated
Very useful in acute severe asthma	Not appropriate in acute setting
Can be used at home and diary produced	Usually unavailable outside of care setting
Useful to detect occupational asthma	Usually unavailable outside of care setting
Not recommended for initial diagnosis	Validated for initial diagnosis of asthma: FEV_1/FVC <70% predicted (in appropriate clinical context)

FEV_1, forced expiratory volume in 1 second; FVC, forced vital capacity.

SPIROMETRY

- Key parameters:
    - FEV_1 – forced expiratory volume in 1 second
        - i.e. how much air is expelled in first second of exhalation;
    - FVC – forced vital capacity
        - i.e. total air expelled from lungs;
    - FEV_1/FVC ratio.

MICRO-facts

FEV_1/FVC ratio
<0.7 in **obstructive** lung disease
>0.8 in **restrictive** lung disease

- Indications:
    - **Asthma**: diagnosis, monitoring, assessment of response to treatment.
    - **COPD**: diagnosis, monitoring, assessment of response to treatment.

Clinical specialties

- Diagnosis of other suspected restrictive or obstructive respiratory conditions, e.g. fibrosing alveolitis, etc.
- Pre-operative assessment of fitness for surgery.
- Preparations:
  - Height, age and sex are recorded.
  - Patient sits upright or is standing.
  - Full inspiration.
  - Rest, no cigarettes and no inhalers/nebulizers for 1 hour before test.

MICRO-facts

Acute asthma features

- Moderate exacerbation
  - PEF <50–75% best or predicted
- Acute severe asthma – any of
  - **S** Sentences incomplete
  - **P** Pulse >110/min
  - **R** Respiration >25/min
  - **50** peak expiratory flow rate (PEFR) 33–50% best or predicted
- Life-threatening asthma – any of
  - **S** Silent chest on auscultation
  - **H** Hypotension
  - **O**ne third PEF (<33% best/predicted)
  - **C** Cyanosis
  - **K** Confusion (!)
  - **S** SaO_2 <92%
  - Exhaustion
  - Arrhythmia
  - Poor respiratory effort
  - Normal $PaCO_2$ (4.7–6.0 kPa)
  - PaO_2 <8 kPa
- Near fatal asthma
  - Raised CO_2
  - Requiring mechanical ventilation with raised inflation pressures

Adapted from BTS guidelines (see below)

MICRO-reference
British Guideline on the Management of Asthma. **Thorax** 2008; 63(Suppl 4): iv1–121.

- Technique:
  - Forced exhalation as hard and fast as possible, continued to full expiration.
- Measurement:
  - Compared with a nomogram based on age, sex and height.
  - Expressed as percentage of predicted value for above parameters.
  - Pattern of FEV_1, FVC and FEV_1/FVC indicative of type of airways disease.

MICRO-facts

- **Obstructive** disease **obstructs** the passage of air out of the lung, therefore FEV_1 is reduced, while FVC is relatively normal. FEV_1/FVC ratio is therefore **low**.
- **Restrictive** disease **restricts** the lung volume, and therefore FVC is **reduced**. FEV_1 may be mildly decreased, but FEV_1/FVC ratio is **normal** or **high**.

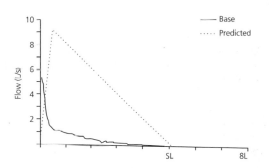

Fig .7.1 Obstructive spirometry. This trace is from a 68-year-old man with chronic obstructive pulmonary disease. He is 197 cm tall. FEV_1, 1.25 (32% predicted); FVC, 4.87 (95% predicted); FEV_1/FVC, 0.26.

- Benefits:
  - Quick, easy, cheap.
  - Broad range of indications including both asthma and COPD.
  - Useful for assessment of treatment response
  - Largely effort independent.
  - Accurate if repeated.
  - More sophisticated than PEF.

- Limitations/problems:
  - Not useful for acute asthma.
  - Only some new models portable.

Asthma

- FEV_1/FVC ratio <0.7 indicates obstructive problem
  - diagnostic in appropriate clinical context.

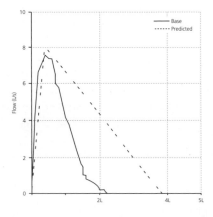

Fig. 7.2 Restrictive spirometry. This trace is from a 53-year-old man with fibrosing alveolitis. He is 167 cm tall. FEV_1, 1.95 (62% predicted); FVC, 2.27 (58% predicted); FEV_1/FVC, 0.86.

Table 7.5 Comparison of obstructive and restrictive patterns on spirometry.

	OBSTRUCTIVE	RESTRICTIVE
Features	$\downarrow\downarrow FEV_1$	$\downarrow FEV_1$
	$\leftrightarrow$ or $\downarrow$ FVC	$\downarrow$ FVC
	$\downarrow\downarrow FEV_1/FVC$	$\leftrightarrow$ or $\uparrow FEV_1/FVC$
Examples	Reversible: asthma	Interstitial: pulmonary fibrosis, sarcoidosis
	Irreversible: COPD	Extrinsic: pneumonia, pleural effusion, tumour
		Chest wall, e.g. kyphoscoliosis, ankylosing spondylitis

COPD, chronic obstructive pulmonary disease; FEV_1, forced expiratory volume in 1 second; FVC, forced vital capacity

Clinical specialties

- Reversibility – indicates asthma
  - assessed before and after inhalation of 400 µg of salbutamol;
  - or before and after 6–8 weeks of inhalation of 200 µg of beclometasone twice daily;
  - or before and after 14 days of 30 mg of oral prednisolone daily;
  - Reversibility: >400 mL improvement in FEV_1.

COPD

- FEV_1/FVC ratio <0.7 indicates obstructive problem
  - diagnostic in appropriate clinical context.
- FEV_1
  - mild airflow obstruction 50–80% predicted;
  - moderate airflow obstruction 30–49% predicted;
  - severe airflow obstruction < 30% predicted.

Restrictive lung disease

- FEV_1/FVC ratio >0.7.
- FVC <80% predicted.

Mixed picture

- FEV_1/FVC ratio < 0.7.
- FVC <80% predicted.

> **MICRO-reference**
> Halpin D. NICE guidance for COPD. **Thorax** 2004; **59**: 181–2.

TRANSFER FACTOR OF CARBON MONOXIDE (T_LCO)

- Measure of diffusion rate of carbon monoxide from alveoli into blood.
- CO has high avidity for haemoglobin, therefore diffuses rapidly.
- Allows estimation of alveolar surface area for gas transfer.
- Transfer factor of carbon monoxide (T_LCO) – gas exchange capacity.
- K_{CO} – CO transfer coefficient, measure of diffusion efficiency.
- Technique:
  - Exhale completely.
  - Complete inhalation of mixture of air containing 10% helium and a trace of CO (>90% vital capacity to be accurate).
  - Hold breath for 10 seconds.
  - Exhaled air collected and analysed.
- **TLCO, KCO is decreased** when lung volume or ability for gas to diffuse is reduced, e.g.:

- COPD, interstitial lung disease – fewer functioning alveoli;
- pulmonary oedema – fewer functioning alveoli;
- anaemia – decreased capacity of blood to receive diffused gas;
- PE – decreased blood supply.

7.4 RESPIRATORY RADIOLOGY

For more information, please refer to Chapter 5, Radiology.

RADIOLOGICAL FINDINGS IN RESPIRATORY MEDICINE

- Pneumonia:
  - Plain chest radiograph
    - consolidation with air bronchogram:
      ○ may persist after patient's symptoms have improved;
    - need not repeat prior to discharge if satisfactory clinical recovery;
    - repeat suggested around 6 weeks after a community acquired pneumonia if:
      ○ persistent symptoms or physical signs;
      ○ if increased risk of underlying malignancy, e.g. smokers or those aged > 50 years.
  - CT scan
    - not required for primary pneumonia;
    - may allow assessment or exclusion of complications, e.g. abscess formation, empyema, underlying malignancy or other interstitial disease processes.

MICRO-reference

Lim WS, Baudouin SV, George RC, Hill AT, Jamieson C, Le Jeune I, et al. BTS guidelines for the management of community acquired pneumonia in adults: update 2009. Thorax 2009; **64** (Suppl 3): iii1–55.

- Pneumothorax:
  - Plain chest radiograph
    - air in pleural cavity, with lung subsequently collapsed and retracting towards the hilum;
    - absent lung markings between lung edge and chest wall;
    - small pneumothorax (less than 20% collapse), with no clinical breathlessness requires no treatment;
    - larger pneumothoraces require aspiration or chest drain insertion;
    - follow-up radiograph needed to ensure complete resolution, e.g. 2 week follow up in patients who do not undergo intervention in primary pneumothorax.

> **MICRO-reference**
> Henry M, Arnold T, Harvey J. BTS guidelines for the management of
> spontaneous pneumothorax. **Thorax** 2003; **58** (Suppl 2): ii39–52.

- Pleural effusion:
  - Plain chest radiograph
    - fluid collection between parietal and visceral pleura;
    - erect radiograph;
      - ○ fluid in lower most part of thorax (dependent on position);
      - ○ loss of costodiaphragmagtic angle with loss of pulmonary and bronchial markings;
      - ○ concave upper border of fluid meniscus;
      - ○ massive effusion would cause a 'white out' of the hemithorax, with possible mediastinal shift if no associated volume loss of the lung.
  - Ultrasound
    - extremely sensitive in detecting even small fluid volumes;
    - can distinguish pleural fluid from pleural masses/thickening;
    - can demonstrate loculation.
  - CT scan with contrast
    - can distinguish benign and malignant pleural disease;
    - can detect extra pleural disease such as lymphadenopathy.
- Tuberculosis:
  - Plain chest radiograph
    - typically shows upper lobe infiltrates with cavitation;
    - may be associated with hilar or paratracheal lymphadenopathy;
    - discrete 1–2 mm nodules may be seen bilaterally throughout lung fields due to haematological spread (miliary TB);
    - may also reveal prior TB infection, such as fibrosis, pleural thickening or calcification.
- Bronchiectasis:
  - Plain chest radiograph
    - may be entirely normal;
    - may also show 'ring shadows' and 'tramlines' – indicates dilated, thickened airways.
  - High-resolution computed tomography (HRCT scans)
    - more than 97% sensitive in detecting bronchiectasis;
    - typically show
      - ○ airway dilatation to lung periphery in affected lobe;
      - ○ bronchial wall thickening;
      - ○ airway appearing larger than its accompanying vessel ('signet ring sign').

- Pulmonary fibrosis:
  - Plain chest radiograph
    - reticulonodular shadowing usually commencing at the bases of the lungs;
    - possible reduction in lung volume;
    - 'shaggy heart' appearance due to lung fibrosis adjacent to the heart borders.
  - HRCT
    - may reveal earlier radiological features of subpleural fibrosis.
    - more sensitive than plain radiographs.
- Emphysema:
  - Plain chest radiograph
    - may be normal;
    - in advanced cases the following may be present:
      - ○ bilaterally hyperinflated lung fields;
      - ○ attenuated vasculature;
      - ○ flattened diaphragm;
      - ○ bullae;
    - Repeated plain radiographs unnecessary unless other pathologies are considered.
- Pulmonary embolus:
  - Plain chest radiograph
    - normal in most cases;
    - if infarction develops the following may be seen:
      - ○ basal collapse and/or segmental consolidation;
      - ○ raised diaphragm;
      - ○ small effusion (40% of cases).
  - Ventilation/perfusion scan (VQ scan)
    - isotope scanning;
    - shows a segmental defect in perfusion with preserved ventilation;
    - mostly superseded by computed tomography pulmonary angiography (CTPA) scans;
    - still conducted when the contrast required for CTPA is contraindicated.
  - CTPA
    - CT scans through the thorax after IV injection of a contrast bolus at high speed;
    - emboli are seen as filling defects in the contrast-filled arteries;
    - highly accurate (>95% sensitivity) even at subsegmental level;
    - usually first-line investigation in suspected PE cases.
  - CT venography
    - an emerging area;
    - combined with CTPA to image the pelvic leg veins simultaneously.

> **MICRO-reference**
> British Thoracic Society guidelines for the management of suspected
> acute pulmonary embolism. **Thorax** 2003; **58**: 470–83.

- Bronchial carcinoma (peripheral):
  - Plain chest radiograph
    - may show lobulated or spiculated masses;
    - associated with hilar gland enlargement, pleural effusion and/or areas of collapse/consolidation.
  - CT
    - aids the assessment of metastatic disease and operability (staging).
- Bronchial carcinoma (central):
  - Plain chest radiograph
    - may show central masses causing:
      - ○ hilar shadow enlargement;
      - ○ narrowing of bronchial lumen;
      - ○ collapse of distal lung;
      - ○ consolidation due to secondary infection.
  - CT
    - aids identification and spread of the tumour;
    - aids treatment decision such as operability.
- Pulmonary metastases:
  - Plain chest radiograph
    - multiple pulmonary nodules may be present.
  - CT
    - more sensitive in detecting lung metastases and lymph node involvement;
    - used in monitoring of response to chemotherapy;
    - CT-PET used to assess locoregional disease for surgical candidates.

7.5 ADDITIONAL RESPIRATORY INVESTIGATIONS

ECG

- Respiratory indications include cor pulmonale and PE.
  - **PE** may be normal but may show:
    - sinus tachycardia;
    - right bundle branch block;
    - right ventricular strain (inverted T wave in V_1–V_4);
    - classical $S_1Q_3T_3$ pattern is rare

- Cor pulmonale:
  - P pulmonale (right atrial hypertrophy giving tall peaked P waves);
  - right axis deviation.

EXERCISE TESTS

- For example, shuttle testing.
- Conducted pre-operatively for high-risk patients to assess functional status.
- Used pre- and post-operatively for lung transplantation and lung volume reduction.
- To assess response to treatments and pulmonary rehabilitation.

INDUCED SPUTUM

- Indications:
  - Suspected deep lung infection, e.g. TB, *Pneumocystis* (*carinii*) *jiroveci* pneumonia (PJP)
  - **and** the patient is unable to produce spontaneous sputum sample, or spontaneous sample negative in context of high clinical suspicion.
- Technique:
  - Nebulizer with 5 mg of salbutamol.
  - Between 5 and 60 mL of hypertonic saline (3%) in a nebulizer.
  - A chest physiotherapist works with patient to breathe and cough.
  - Sputum is produced.
  - **Microbiology,** e.g. microscopy culture and sensitivity, polymerase chain reaction (PCR) for viruses, immunofluorescence, e.g. for PJP, auramine phenol stain for acid-fast bacilli, TB culture, etc.

BRONCHOSCOPY

- Indications include masses on imaging (i.e. suspected cancer), haemoptysis, cough, wheeze, stridor, suspected inhaled foreign body, transbronchial biopsy for interstitial disease and therapeutic intervention (e.g. insertion of stents).
- Allows visualization of tissue.
- Samples:
  - In the form of washings, brushings, mucosal biopsies or transbronchial biopsy.
  - **Microbiology,** e.g. microscopy, culture and sensitivity (MC&S), PCR for viruses, immunofluorescence, e.g. for PJP, auramine phenol stain for acid-fast bacilli, TB culture, etc.
  - **Histology/cytology** to investigate suspected cancer and decide on therapy.

- Complications:
  - pneumothorax;
  - pneumonia;
  - haemorrhage.

Micro-print
Other respiratory investigations:

- α1-Antitrypsin blood test. Deficiency increases risk of emphysema + COPD at an earlier age, +/- lung irritant exposure.
- Sputum eosinophil count: >2% indicates asthma. ↑sensitivity, moderate specificity
- Sweat test for cystic fibrosis (CF). Pilocarpine ionophoresis stimulates sweat production which is analysed. A positive result is >60 mmol/L of chloride. A level of 40–60 mmol/L is suggestive, but not diagnostic, of CF. Sweat sodium level is less reliable and should be interpreted in context of chloride level; however, >90 mmol/L suggests CF.
- Polysomnography. To diagnose obstructive sleep apnoea (OSA) and other related breathing disorders. Parameters include pulse oximetry, ECG, nasal/oral air flow, EEG, continuous video monitoring, sound recordings, surface electromyography and electrooculography.

Gastrointestinal medicine

8.1 BLOOD TESTS

- Full blood count (FBC):
    - Microcytic anaemia may be due to iron deficiency in which there may be an iron absorption abnormality (see Chapter 1, Haematology) or a source of chronic bleeding.
    - Macrocytic anaemia may be due to vitamin B_{12} or folate deficiency (see Chapter 1, Haematology).
    - Normocytic normochromic anaemia may be an anaemia of chronic disease or due to acute blood loss, e.g. via a peptic or duodenal ulcer.
    - Apparent polycythaemia may be due to dehydration.
    - Neutrophilia may be due to bacterial infection or inflammation, e.g. inflammatory bowel disease or diverticulosis
    - Reactive thrombocytosis may be secondary to infection, inflammation, bleeding or malignancy.
- Urea and electrolytes (U + E):
    - In significant gastrointestinal bleeds a difference in urea and creatinine can be found, with urea significantly raised (blood is high in protein and so once metabolized in the gastrointestinal (GI) tract urea rises).
    - Sepsis anywhere within the body, including the GI tract, may precipitate acute renal failure, especially if the patient is jaundiced.
- Serum amylase:
    - High levels (>5 times normal) indicate acute pancreatitis.
    - Raised levels, but below five times the normal, can occur in many causes of an acute abdomen and are not diagnostic of pancreatitis.
    - Mildly raised levels can also occur in chronic pancreatitis.
- Acute-phase reactants (erythrocyte sedimentation rate (ESR) and C-reactive protein (CRP)):

- These are raised in cases of inflammation (e.g. inflammatory bowel disease) and/or infections.
- Serum pregnancy test.

MICRO-facts

Pregnancy or ectopic pregnancies should be excluded in the presentation of an acute surgical abdomen in any woman of child-bearing age.

- Glucose:
  - Diabetic ketoacidosis must be excluded in patients presenting with an acute abdomen.
- Calcium levels:
  - Hypercalcaemia may cause constipation.
  - May cause abdominal pain by direct effect on bowel motility, or from renal calculi.
- Thyroid function tests:
  - Hypothyroidism may cause constipation, whereas hyperthyroidism may precipitate diarrhoea.
- Blood cultures:
  - These are required if septicaemia is suspected.
- Antibodies:
  - Pernicious anaemia may be indicated by the presence of:
    - anti-parietal cell antibody;
    - anti-intrinsic factor antibody.
  - Coeliac disease may be indicated by the presence of:
    - anti-tissue transglutaminase antibody – first-line screening test;
    - anti-endomysial antibody (IgA) – high sensitivity and specificity – and is useful if anti-tissue transglutaminase antibody test result is equivocal;
    - anti-reticulin antibody – highly sensitive but not so specific, and also seen in other GI conditions (e.g. Crohn's disease);
    - Anti-gliadin antibody.

8.2 DETAILED LIVER ASSESSMENT (NON-INVASIVE LIVER SCREEN)

Abnormalities are often found in routine liver function tests (LFTs) (see Chapter 2, Clinical chemistry). A non-invasive liver screen comprises a wide range of tests designed to detect the most common causes of liver dysfunction. Should these tests not lead to a diagnosis, magnetic resonance imaging (MRI) or liver biopsy may be considered.

Clinical specialties

- Full liver function tests (LFTs):
  - This will include some of the less commonly measured LFTs, e.g. gamma-glutamyl transpeptidase (γ-GT/GGT), which may give important information to indicate the patient's diagnosis.
- Coagulation screen:
  - Prothrombin time (PT) in particular is a sensitive marker of hepatic synthetic dysfunction as the liver produces clotting factors. Prolonged PT would indicate poor liver function.
- Iron profile:
  - Raised ferritin and iron with a low total iron-binding capacity (TIBC) would suggest haemochromatosis (see Chapter 1, Haematology).
- Caeruloplasmin:
  - The carrier protein for copper in serum. This is low in Wilson's disease, which is characterized by systemic copper excess, deposition in the liver and damage to the organ.
- Autoantibodies:
  - To detect autoimmune hepatitis.
  - Anti-nuclear antibody (ANA).
  - Anti-liver/kidney microsomal-1 (LKM-1) antibody.
  - Anti-smooth muscle antibody.
  - Anti-mitochondrial (AMA) antibody – raised in primary biliary cirrhosis.
- α1-Antitrypsin:
  - Deficiency may lead to liver dysfunction as well as chronic obstructive pulmonary disease (COPD) in early life.
- α-Fetoprotein (AFP) – tumour marker:
  - Elevated levels suggest hepatocellular carcinoma.
  - May also be raised in germ cell (i.e. testicular/ovarian) tumours, hepatitis, pregnancy and cirrhosis.
  - Note that tumour markers are not diagnostic, and further investigations would be required to prove a diagnosis.
- Viral hepatitis screen:
  - Hep A immunoglobulin (Ig) M (acute infection).
  - Hep E serology (IgM acute).
  - Hep B sAg/Ab (surface antigen and antibody) – acute/previous infection.
  - Hep C Ab – antibody and polymerase chain reaction (PCR) for viral RNA.
  - Cytomegalovirus (CMV) and Epstein–Barr Virus (EBV) serology tests.
- Ultrasound of liver:
  - A non-invasive test.
  - Will demonstrate many different liver pathologies.

8.3 OTHER COMMON GASTROINTESTINAL INVESTIGATIONS

URINE SAMPLES

- Increased bilirubin and decreased urobilinogen may indicate biliary obstruction.
- A urinary pregnancy test is often conducted in females presenting with iliac fossa pain, to rule out an ectopic pregnancy.

STOOL SAMPLES

- Cultures and microscopy should always be performed when diarrhoea is present to identify any infective causes.
- Fat content of stool samples occasionally needs to be confirmed in the presence of steatorrhoea in suspected fat malabsorption. This is often avoided by breath analysis using radiolabelled fat load.
- Faecal occult blood tests may also be conducted as part of a screening process for colorectal cancers, using a high sensitivity method to detect blood in the stool sample.

BREATH TESTS

- Hydrogen breath tests:
    - These are often used as a screening test for bacterial overgrowth.
    - Oral lactulose or glucose is metabolized by bacteria with production of hydrogen.
    - An early rise in hydrogen indicates either bacterial overgrowth in the upper small bowel or rapid transit of the colon, where bacteria are inevitably present.
- ^{14}C breath test (urease breath test):
    - Radioactively labelled carbon bile salts given by mouth to patient.
    - Bacteria deconjugate the bile salts and release the radioactive carbon, appearing in the breath as $^{14}CO_2$.
    - An early rise in $^{14}CO_2$ indicates either bacterial overgrowth in the upper small bowel or rapid transit of the colon, where bacteria are inevitably present.
    - Used in detection of *Helicobacter pylori* infection of the stomach.

24-HOUR INTRALUMINAL pH MONITORING

- This involves the positioning of a pH-sensitive probe in the lower oesophagus via the nose.
- Is used for the identification of reflux episodes (pH < 4), with a record of the correlation of the episodes with the patient's symptoms.

- Note that normal subjects can have brief episodes of pH < 4.
- This investigation is often conducted alongside manometry.

MANOMETRY

- A fluid-filled catheter is passed through the nose, into the oesophagus.
- Any changes in pressure are transmitted up the fluid-filled column and detected.
- It is used for motility problems, e.g. achalasia.

ENDOSCOPY TYPES

- Oesophagogastroduodenoscopy (OGD):
    - High diagnostic accuracy, being the investigation of choice in upper GI disorders.
    - Easy access, allowing therapeutic interventions (e.g. injection of ulcers with adrenaline, oesphageal stenting / balloon dilatation) and diagnostic biopsies (e.g. biopsy of gastric mucosa).
    - The patient is fasted overnight, and the procedure may be carried out as an outpatient.
    - It is contraindicated in:
        - severe COPD;
        - recent myocardial infarction;
        - instability of atlanto-axial joint.
    - Complications include perforation and aspiration pneumonia.

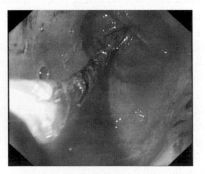

Fig. 8.1 Oesophagogastroduodenoscopy image of the pylorus with a deflated balloon passed through it. Courtesy of Mr Kirtik Patel, Consultant Upper GI and Bariatric Surgeon, Northern General Hospital, Sheffield.

- Colonoscopy:
    - Allows good visualization of the colon and terminal ileum.
    - Indications include:
        - suspected inflammatory bowel disease;
        - polyp follow-up;

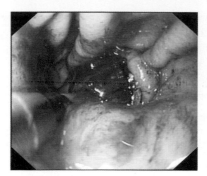

Fig. 8.2 Oesophagogastroduodenoscopy image of balloon dilatation of a pyloric stricture. Courtesy of Mr Kirtik Patel, Consultant Upper GI and Bariatric Surgeon, Northern General Hospital, Sheffield.

  – anaemia with or without rectal bleeding;
  – unexplained weight loss;
  – chronic diarrhoea.
- Biopsies can be obtained and polyps removed.
- Bowel preparation (including low residue diet and laxatives) needed prior to investigation.
- Complications include perforation or haemorrhage following biopsy or polypectomy.

MICRO-refrence
WHO guidelines for colorectal cancer. http://www.who.int/cancer/detection/colorectalcancer/en/ (accessed 05/04/11).

- Sigmoidoscopy:
  - This allows visualization of the rectum and distal colon.
  - It is often used as a screening procedure prior to a full colonoscopy
  - It can be done in preference to a full colonoscopy in patients having an active flare of ulcerative colitis or Crohn's disease to avoid a perforation of the colon.
- Capsule endoscopy:
  - A camera in a capsule is swallowed to allow visualization of GI tract that cannot be visualized by other endoscopy methods, e.g. proximal small bowel.
  - A routine 'test' empty capsule is often swallowed prior to the camera capsule in order to ensure there is no stricture within the bowel, to ensure that when the camera capsule is swallowed, it will not get blocked.

Clinical specialties

MICRO-refrence
NICE interventional procedures overview. Wireless capsule endoscopy (Jan 2004). http://www.nice.org.uk/guidance/index.jsp?action = download&o = 31216 (accessed 05/04/11).

SOME USES OF ENDOSCOPY

Endoscopy does not allow therapeutic intervention or biopsies to be taken but it allows the following to be conducted.

- Rapid urease test:
  - Also known as CLO (*Campylobacter*-like organism) test.
  - Gastric biopsies taken from endoscopy are added to a urea solution containing phenol.
  - If *Helicobacter pylori* is present, the urease enzyme splits the urea, releasing ammonia and raising the pH, causing a rapid colour change.
- Biopsy/histology:
  - *H. pylori* may be detected histologically on routine (Giemsa) stained sections of gastric mucosa.
  - Jejunal biopsy is often conducted to aid the diagnosis of coeliac disease, where the histological appearance of flattened mucosa with sub-total villous atrophy and proliferation of the crypts of Lieberkuhn are diagnostic.
  - A smear of jejunal juice or mucosal impression may aid diagnosis of *Giardia lamblia.*
  - Intestinal biopsy may show periodic acid–Schiff (PAS)-positive macrophages in Whipple's disease.
  - Rectal and colonic biopsies are obtainable for histological examination of suspicious lesions.
- Gram-stain and culture:
  - This allows sensitivities to antibiotics to be ascertained, if necessary.

MICRO-refrence
BSG (British Society of Gastroenterology) Guidelines in Gastroenterology. May 2005. http://www.bsg.org.uk/pdf_word_docs/iron_def.pdf (accessed 05/04/11).

RADIOLOGY

For more information, please refer to Chapter 5, Radiology.

Hiatus hernia

- Erect chest radiograph:
  - hiatus hernia would show a soft-tissue mass behind the cardiac shadow;
- Barium swallow:
  - a rolling hiatus hernia will have its gastro-oesophageal junction below the diaphragm, with the stomach herniating alongside the oesophagus;
  - a sliding hiatus hernia will have its gastro-oesophageal junction above the diaphragm.

Gastric ulcers

- OGD is the gold standard.
- Erect chest radiograph:
  - may reveal pneumoperitoneum as a complication of perforated ulcers.
- Barium meal:
  - a pool of barium contrast may collect within the ulcer crater, with the mucosal folds projecting into the ulcer.
- CT:
  - may show a pneumoperitoneum if perforated ulcer.

Crohn's disease

- Small bowel study:
  - deep ulceration creating a 'rose thorn' effect;
  - cobblestone appearance of the mucosa due to ulcers separated by areas of oedema;
  - thickened and rigid bowel wall causing separation of the small bowel loops;
  - stricture formation due to oedema and fibrosis, typically in terminal ileum.

Gallstones

- Abdominal radiographs:
  - 10% of calculi are visible as they are radio-opaque.
- Ultrasound:
  - first-line investigation of choice for assessment of the hepatobiliary tree;
  - gallstones appear as echogenic areas casting an acoustic shadow;
  - gallbladder wall thickening in acute cholecystitis;
  - the common bile duct may also be assessed – dilatation suggests a distal blockage, most commonly a calculus;
  - magnetic resonance cholangiopancreatography (MRCP) is excellent for detecting bile duct stones.

Clinical specialties

Acute pancreatitis

- Plain radiographs:
  - chest radiograph may show reactive pleural effusion (more prominent on the left side), due to the high amylase levels;
  - abdominal radiographs may show gallstones (a cause of the pancreatitis), absence of gas in the abdomen, or an ileus. Rarely, a 'sentinel loop' of bowel may be apparent in the pancreatic region, and calcification of the pancreas may be present in chronic pancreatitis with acute exacerbation.
- Ultrasound:
  - may not be helpful if there is significant bowel distension, causing obscuration of the pancreas by bowel gas;
  - pancreas may be seen as normal, or may be enlarged and oedematous. It is most important to identify gallstones as a potential cause of the pancreatitis;
  - pancreatic duct and/or common bile duct may be dilated;
  - pseudocyst formation may be seen, most commonly in the lesser sac.
- CT:
  - outlines the oedematous, inflamed pancreas;
  - should only be performed for the identification of complications of pancreatitis, such as necrosis, haemorrhage, pseudocysts and pseudoaneurysm formation.

Pancreatic carcinoma

- Ultrasound:
  - pancreatic and bile ducts may be dilated;
  - gallbladder may be dilated;
  - there may be associated liver metastases or ascites;
  - there may be a focal pancreatic enlargement with a hypoechoic mass.
- CT scan:
  - the investigation of choice;
  - invasion of the carcinoma into the mesenteric vessels may be apparent, along with metastases to other organs (e.g. liver).
- MRI:
  - will show a reduced signal from the pancreatic mass on a T_1 sequence scan.
- Endoscopic retrograde cholangiopancreatography (ERCP):
  - may show irregular ductal obstruction;
  - only used when ultrasound or computed tomography (CT) do not provide a confirmed diagnosis.

LAPAROSCOPY

- This is conducted as a diagnostic tool, prior to proceeding with the planned surgery to ensure alternative or simultaneous pathology is not found.

MICRO-print
Further specific radiology

- Barium swallow
    - Involves a contrast agent of barium sulphate (unless perforation of GI tract is suspected, when a water-soluble contrast agent is used instead, such as gastrograffin).
    - Indications include dysphagia and gastro-oesophageal reflux.
    - Fluoroscopy is used to visualize the passing of contrast agent down the oesophagus looking for motility or structural abnormalities.
    - Often substituted by conducting oesophagoscopy which allows direct visualization with ability to obtain histology and cytological proof of carcinomas when appropriate.
- Barium follow-through study
    - Conducted by observing 200–300 mL of barium contrast as it transits through the small bowel, with intermittent screening at regular intervals until it reaches the large bowel.
- Barium meal
    - Having fasted overnight, the patient is given a double contrast of gas (via oral effervescent powder) followed by a barium contrast drink.
    - Usually conducted when OGD not feasible.
    - Allows the viewing of the GI tract with fluoroscopy, especially indicated with suspected stomach pathology such as gastric outlet obstruction. Only used when OGD cannot be performed.
- Barium enema
    - Involves cleaning of the colon using laxatives, followed by barium and air administered per rectum.
    - Mainly indicated when there is a change in bowel habit.
    - Contraindicated in pseudomembranous colitis, toxic megacolon and recent radiotherapy or full bowel thickness biopsy.
    - Complications include bowel perforation (rare).
    - Usually due to a failed colonoscopy or patient choice.
    - Often substituted by conducting colonoscopy which allows direct visualization with ability to obtain histology and cytological proof of lesions via biopsy and removal of polyps when appropriate.

continued...

Clinical specialties

continued...

- ERCP (endoscopic retrograde cholangiopancreatography)
  - Indicated for removal of gallstones or stenting of the common bile duct in obstructive jaundice. Also for investigation of suspected pancreatic malignancy.
  - Endoscope passed orally in prone position.
  - Cannulation of the ampulla of Vater allows injection of contrast allowing visualization of the pancreatic and bile ducts.
  - Sphincter of Oddi can be cut to facilitate removal of stones and stent insertion. Vitamin K often required prior to procedure to prevent haemorrhage from this sphincterotomy.
  - Complications include bleeding, acute pancreatitis and duodenal perforation.
- MRCP
  - Alternative non-invasive technique for imaging the biliary system.
- Coeliac axis and mesenteric angiography
  - Contrast agent injected into the superior and/or inferior mesenteric arteries via femoral artery catheter. Used to pinpoint the source of acute haemorrhage of the small or large bowel.

9 Genitourinary and renal medicine

9.1 BLOOD TESTS

- Full blood count (FBC):
    - There may be decreased haemoglobin levels in chronic renal failure and blood loss.
    - Renal tumours or cysts may produce excess erythropoietin resulting in polycythaemia.
    - Leucocytosis is commonly found in acute renal failure.
    - Leucopenia and thrombocytopenia may suggest systemic lupus erythematosus (SLE).

> **MICRO-facts**
>
> Note that the GFR may fall significantly before urea or creatinine levels fall outside of their reference range.
>
> A patient with severe renal disease may still have urea and creatinine levels within the normal range.

- Urea and electrolytes (U + E) (see Chapter 2, Clinical chemistry). Note that is it more important to analyse the trend of these results than the isolated results:
    - Urea levels, as a crude indicator of renal function, may be increased in renal disease, high protein intake and fever.
    - Creatinine, as an indicator of renal function, may be increased in all types of renal disease.
    - Albumin may decrease in nephrotic syndrome, but may increase in dehydration.
    - The estimated glomerular filtration rate (eGFR) is an accurate measurement for renal function, allowing for differences in muscle mass, age, sex and race, and is decreased in renal failure.
    - Sodium and potassium levels may be deranged in renal disease, along with an increased anion gap.

- Arterial blood gases:
  - Metabolic acidosis is commonly found in renal failure (e.g. renal tubular necrosis giving a normal anion gap); respiratory compensation by hyperventilation may occur.
- Blood glucose:
  - This may be raised, indicating diabetes mellitus and its possible renal complications.
- Erythrocyte sedimentation rate (ESR):
  - Infection, renal cell carcinoma, vasculitis and retroperitoneal fibrosis may all elevate the ESR.
- Urate (uric acid):
  - Increased urate will increase the risk of gout and renal/urinary calculi and can lead to chronic renal failure due to urate nephropathy.
  - Note that urate levels may be low or normal during an acute attack of gout.
- Calcium levels:
  - Calcium is often requested with the uric acid levels.
  - Hypercalcaemia may be another cause of renal calculi or renal damage causing polyuria and/or polydipsia.
- Prostate-specific antigen (PSA):
  - Prostatic carcinoma and metastatic disease lead to increased levels of PSA. A small rise may also be seen in prostatic hyperplasia.
  - Note that levels must be compared to age-specific reference ranges.

MICRO-facts

Causes of a raised PSA include:

- prostate carcinoma;
- instrumentation of prostate (including urinary catheterization);
- urinary tract infection;
- recent ejaculation.

- α-Fetoprotein (α-FP):
  - This is a marker for testicular tumours.
  - Note that this also has good specificity for hepatocellular carcinoma; and when testing for testicular tumours, it is advisable to test for both α-FP and β-human chorionic gonadotrophin (β-hCG).
- β-hCG:
  - In men, this may be used as a marker for testicular tumours, including seminomas.
- Other serum tests:
  - Antinuclear antibody (ANA) may be present in significant titre in systemic lupus erythematosus.

- Complement 3 (C3) and complement 4 (C4) levels may be lowered in systemic lupus erythematosus.
- Anti-neutrophil cytoplasmic antibodies (ANCA) are seen as markers for vasculitides, such as Wegener's granulomatosis, involving the kidney, with or without signs of systemic disease.
- Anti-glomerular basement membrane (anti-GBM) is found to be positive in Goodpasture's syndrome.
- Hepatitis B surface antigen – infection with hepatitis B can cause membranous nephropathy or polyarteritis nodosa (PAN).
- Hepatitis C antibody – infection with hepatitis C can cause cryoglobulinaemia.
- HIV antibody – infection with HIV can cause renal damage (HIV-associated glomerulonephritis).
- Cryoglobulins – these are present in cryoglobulinaemia.

9.2 URINE ANALYSIS

URINE COLLECTION

There are several urine sample collection methods. Urine may be collected as one-off sample collections, or over a period of 24 hours (e.g. to measure 24 hour urine protein, or to calculate creatinine clearance).

- Clean-catch midstream urine (MSU):
  - Advantages
    - it flushes contaminating cells and microbes from the outer urethra prior to collection by discarding first half of bladder volume.
  - Disadvantages
    - patients often find it difficult to comply with the rules of discarding the primary volume of urine and catching the second;
    - requires the patient to clean their external urethra prior to collection.
- Random catch:
  - Advantages
    - easy for patients to comply with the collection technique and it can be done any time of day with no precautions regarding contamination.
  - Disadvantages
    - sample may be dilute, isotonic or hypertonic and may contain white cells, bacteria and squamous epithelium as contaminants;
    - in females, the specimen may contain vaginal contaminants such as trichomonads, yeasts, and, during menses, red cells.
- Early-morning collection:
  - Advantages
    - usually hypertonic and reflects the ability of the kidney to concentrate urine during dehydration which occurs overnight.

Clinical specialties

- Disadvantages
  - patient is required to collect urine prior to ingesting any fluids in the morning.
- 'In/out' catheterization via the urethra:
  - Advantages
    - allows sample to be obtained from comatose or confused patients.
  - Disadvantages
    - risks introducing infection and traumatizing the urethra and bladder, thus producing iatrogenic infection or haematuria.
- Catheter sample of urine (CSU):
  - Advantages
    - simple to take from a catheterized patient.
  - Disadvantages
    - haematuria and proteinuria may be found with catheter samples (iatrogenic);
    - microbial colonization of long-term catheters is usual. Act on positive bacterial cultures only if clinical features of infection.
- Suprapubic transabdominal needle aspiration of the bladder:
  - Advantages
    - when done under ideal conditions, provides the purest sampling of bladder urine;
    - a good method for infants and small children.
  - Disadvantages
    - invasive, with risk of producing iatrogenic infection or haematuria;
    - may cause pain/ discomfort;
    - only very rarely performed in adults.

URINE DIPSTICK TESTING

Table 9.1 Urine dipstick interpretation.

DIPSTICK TESTS	CONSEQUENCE OF ABNORMAL RESULT
pH	Alkaline urine predisposes to urinary calculi Alkalotic urine suggests infection with an ammonia splitting organism such as *Proteus mirabilis*
Protein	May occur in many circumstances, including posture/ orthostasis (especially in morning), fever, UTI, nephritic syndrome, nephritis, glomerulonephritis, diabetes, exercise and pregnancy Note that Bence–Jones protein is not detected by dipstick

(Continued)

Table 9.1 (*Continued*)

DIPSTICK TESTS	CONSEQUENCE OF ABNORMAL RESULT
Glucose	Glucose in urine increases with age. Its presence suggests, but is not diagnostic of, diabetes
Blood	If positive, the urine must be sent for microscopy to confirm presence of red cells, as the dipstick also detects haemoglobin Main causes include infection, stones, trauma, tumours or haemoglobinopathies
Nitrites	Nitrites are produced by Gram-negative bacteria such as *E. coli*, due to the conversion of nitrates to nitrites
Leucocytes	May be increased due to inflammation in the kidneys or urinary tract (e.g. UTI, stones, trauma), neoplasms, or infection of urinary tract or surrounding structures (e.g. prostatitis)
Specific gravity	Gives a vague guide to the concentration of urine, but this is not 100% reliable; urine osmolality is gold standard
β-hCG	Conducted using specific pregnancy urine sticks Usually shows positive result within 12 days of conception

β-hCG, β-human chorionic gonadotrophin; UTI, urinary tract infection.

URINE MICROSCOPY

Table 9.2 Urine microscopy interpretation.

MICROSCOPY TESTS	CONSEQUENCE OF ABNORMAL RESULT
White cells	>10 per mm^2 is significant May be due to inflammation of the kidneys or urinary tract (e.g. UTI, stones, trauma), neoplasms, or infection of surrounding structures (e.g. prostatitis)
Bacteria	Highly suggestive of a UTI Gram staining may aid the identification of the pathogen Sample culturing required for complete identification of pathogen

(*Continued*)

Clinical specialties

Table 9.2 (*Continued*)

MICROSCOPY TESTS	CONSEQUENCE OF ABNORMAL RESULT
Red cells	>2 per mm^2 is abnormal With proteinuria suggests glomerular pathology Without proteinuria suggests a tumour or stones With nitrites/white cells: likely to be UTI or pyelonephritis With no red cells, but positive on dipstick, then it is suggestive of haemoglobinuria, due to haemolytic anaemia or rhabdomyolysis
Casts	Red cell casts may be found in glomerulonephritis or malignant hypertension Granular casts may be found in acute tubular necrosis, glomerulonephritis or interstitial nephritis White cell casts may be found in pyelonephritis or acute interstitial nephritis

URINE CULTURE AND SENSITIVITY

See Chapter 4, Microbiology, for more information.
- Samples that are sent for microscopy are routinely cultured over 48 hours, with a positive culture producing $>100\,000$ colony-forming units/mL.
- The sample is then re-cultured to detect which antibiotic(s) the pathogens are sensitive to.
- Mixed cultures often indicate contamination.

URINE BIOCHEMISTRY

See Chapter 2, Clinical chemistry, for more information.
- Sodium concentration is helpful in acute renal failure.
  - Low sodium (<20 mmol/L) suggests hypoperfusion (e.g. hypovolaemia).
  - High sodium (>30 mmol/L) suggests acute tubular necrosis.
- Urine osmolality gives an accurate measure of concentration of urine.
- 24 hour protein allows the measurement of protein loss.
- Creatinine clearance allows estimation of the glomerular filtration rate (GFR). This is done by assessing the 24 hour urine collection to calculate the amount of creatinine excreted per minute.

9.3 OTHER COMMON GENITOURINARY AND RENAL INVESTIGATIONS

GENITOURINARY AND RENAL RADIOLOGY

For more information, please refer to Chapter 5, Radiology.

Urinary tract calculi
- Plain radiographs (e.g. KUB – kidney, ureter, bladder film):
  - This may identify calculi in the distribution of the kidneys, ureters and bladder.
  - Calculi may be missed if they overlie bony structures, if hidden behind overlying gas and faecal material, or may be confused with phleboliths and/or arterial calcification.
  - Good for the follow up of patients with known calculi to assess the 'stone status'.
- Intravenous urogram (IVU):
  - Filling defects may be visualized due to obstruction/delayed excretion of contrast, with possible distortion in the pelvic calyces or ureters.
  - Mainly replaced by contrast CT-IVU.
- Ultrasound scan:
  - Accurate overview of the kidneys, allowing the detection of calculi and their complications such as hydronephrosis.
  - Used to guide nephrostomy insertion due to obstructive stone disease.
- Non-contrast CT KUB:
  - Excellent detection of ureteric calculi, up to 99% sensitivity for calculi ≥ 1 mm in size.

Polycystic kidney disease (PKD)
- Ultrasound:
  - This allows measurement of renal size and the number and distribution of cysts.
  - PKD may also be diagnosed antenatally using ultrasound.
- CT or magnetic resonance imaging (MRI):
  - Sharp, well-delineated lesions may be seen and characterized.

Renal artery stenosis
- Ultrasound:
  - Small kidneys with altered Doppler flow in the renal artery.
  - Technically challenging.
- IVU:
  - May be entirely normal.
  - May show delayed uptake of contrast and decreased pole to pole kidney diameter.

- MRI:
  - This is the investigation of choice.
  - Non-invasive visualization of stenosis using magnetic resonance angiography (MRA).
- Renal arteriography:
  - Shows stenosis using contrast injected directly into renal arteries, following selective catheterization of the renal arteries.
  - Allows localization of the stenosis within the artery and potential treatment by angioplasty or stenting.

Renal carcinoma

- Ultrasound:
  - Allows differentiation between solid tumours and benign cysts.
  - Ultrasound-guided biopsy possible.
- CT/MRI:
  - Allows accurate staging of the primary mass by assessing size, enhancement characteristics as well as locoregional and metastatic disease.

Urinary incontinence

- Urodynamic studies, e.g. using cystography:
  - Measurements of micturating pressures inside the bladder in comparison to the abdominal pressure (measured by rectal catheter). Helps differentiate between stress and urge incontinence.
  - Urinary flow rate in a micturating cystogram measured for further diagnosis of the pathophysiological cause of incontinence.

Prostatic enlargement

- Plain radiograph:
  - Prostatic calcification and calculi common, seen above the symphysis pubis.
  - Sclerotic bone lesions may be seen if prostate carcinoma metastases are present.
- Transrectal ultrasound:
  - Assesses size and location of masses, with ability to biopsy suspicious areas.
  - Assessment of local involvement and invasion possible, prostatic size, and shape also determined to help stage the tumour.
- MRI:
  - Allows more accurate staging. It is conducted when radical prostatectomy is being considered to assess for extracapsular spread and nodal metastases.
- Bone scan/ isotope scan:
  - 'Hot spots', indicate bony metastasic disease.

- Note that false positives are common from osteoarthritis and old fractures.

Testicular enlargement/masses

- Ultrasound:
  - Allows evaluation of the testes and other scrotal structures.

10 Neurology

10.1 BLOOD TESTS

- Full blood count (FBC):
  - Anaemia may cause non-specific neurological symptoms such as syncope and weakness, but may also be a sign of chronic disease.
  - Polycythaemia may predispose to strokes.
- White cell count (WCC):
  - Neutrophilia may be present in infection, such as meningitis.
  - Neutropenia may be present in leukaemias, lymphomas and multiple myeloma.
  - Lymphocytosis may indicate viral infections, such as transverse myelitis or Guillian–Barré syndrome.
- Urea and electrolytes (U + E):
  - Electrolyte disturbances, such as hypocalcaemia, may predispose to peripheral neuropathies, confusion, fits and weakness.
  - Some neurological pathologies may predispose to electrolyte disturbances such as: syndrome of inappropriate antidiuretic hormone secretion (SIADH) from intracranial lesions (see Chapter 2, Clinical chemistry).
- Glucose:
  - Hyperglycaemia can cause neuropathies and comas.
  - Hypoglycaemia can cause confusion, comas and focal neurological signs.
- Creatine kinase (CK):
  - High levels may be present in myopathies such as dystrophies and myositis.
- Liver function tests (LFTs):
  - Liver disease may cause confusion, tremors and neuropathy.
- Thyroid function tests:
  - Low thyroid hormone may be a cause of confusion, hyporeflexia, neuropathy and dementia.
  - Thyrotoxicosis is a cause of tremors, confusion and hyperreflexia.

- Blood cultures:
  - Bacterial infections can cause a range of conditions including meningitis, cerebral abscesses and septicaemia.
  - Bacterial infection is implicated in the pathogenesis of conditions such as Guillian–Barré syndrome (*Campylobacter jejuni*).
- Erythrocyte sedimentation rate (ESR) and C-reactive protein (CRP):
  - Markers of inflammation and infection, useful in relevant conditions (e.g. systemic lupus erythematosus (SLE) and giant cell arteritis which can cause nerve infarction, confusion and seizures).
- Folate and vitamin B_{12}:
  - Deficiencies can lead to dementia or peripheral neuropathies.
- Coagulation tests:
  - May show an inherited predisposition to thrombosis.
- Immunology autoantibodies:
  - Acetylcholine receptor antibodies are associated with myasthenia gravis.
  - Antinuclear antibody (ANA) and anti-double stranded DNA (anti-dsDNA) are associated with SLE – a cause of many neurological symptoms such as fits, confusion, neuropathy and aseptic meningitis.

10.2 OTHER COMMON NEUROLOGY INVESTIGATIONS

LUMBAR PUNCTURE

In practice, a lumbar puncture is rarely performed in patients with systemic sepsis as the risk of introducing infection into the CSF and beyond outweighs the benefits. Accordingly, treatment is started empirically and a lumbar puncture may be performed after clinical improvement.

- Indications:
  - Suspected meningitis/encephalitis or other central nervous system (CNS) infections.
  - Suspected subarachnoid haemorrhage.
  - Suspected multiple sclerosis.
- Contraindications:
  - Signs of raised intracranial pressure.
  - Focal neurological signs.
  - Respiratory distress.
  - Significant clotting abnormalities.

- Procedure:
  - A spinal needle is inserted in between the spinous processes of lumbar vertebrae (usually L3–4) into the subarachnoid space.
  - Cerebrospinal fluid (CSF) pressure is measured with a manometer.
  - CSF is then drained and sent for analysis.
- Tests:
  - Cell count (with differential), protein, glucose.
  - Microscopy culture and sensitivity.
  - Polymerase chain reaction (PCR):
    - specific assays to assess for the presence of common CNS pathogens;
    - enterovirus;
    - herpes simplex virus (HSV) types 1 and 2;
    - varicella zoster virus (VZV);
    - *Neisseria meningitidis*;
    - *Streptococcus pneumoniae*.
  - Xanthochromia:
    - a breakdown product of red blood cells;
    - raised 12 hours after a subarachnoid haemorrhage, levels may still be elevated for 2 weeks after the event.
  - Oligoclonal bands:
    - immunoglobulin within the CSF;
    - often, but not always found in patients with multiple sclerosis;
    - needs a paired serum sample sending to check for oligoclonal bands in the blood.
  - **Serum glucose**: if CSF glucose less than 40% serum glucose, suggests bacterial meningitis.

MICRO-facts

CSF changes in meningitis

	VIRAL	BACTERIAL	TB
WCC	↑ Lymphocytes	↑ Neutrophils	↑ Lymphocytes
Glucose	Normal/↓	↓↓	↓↓↓
Protein	Normal/↑	↑↑	↑↑↑

WCC, white cell count.

NEURORADIOLOGY

For more information, please refer to Chapter 5, Radiology.

Headache following head trauma

- Plain skull radiograph:
  - Fractures of the skull vault or base. Now rarely used.
- CT head:
  - Bone window allows visualization of any fractures.
  - Blood collections in the subdural space have a concave inner border.
  - Blood collections in the extradural space have a convex inner border.
  - Blood in cisterns, fissures or ventricles indicates a subarachnoid bleed, often due to trauma, but also may be due to spontaneous ruptured aneurysms.

Table 10.1 Appearances of haemorrhage on head CT over time.

PHASE	DENSITY	APPEARANCE ON CT RELATIVE TO BRAIN PARENCHYMA
Acute	Hyperdense	Bright
7–10 days	Isodense	Difficult to distinguish
21–30 days	Hypodense	Dark

Stroke/transient ischaemic attack

- CT scans:
  - Often remains normal in the early stages, but some substantial infarcts may be seen within the first 24 hours.
  - Acute clot may be visible as a 'hyperdense artery' sign.
  - Haemorrhagic strokes (15%) represented by hyperdense (bright white) areas, the thalamus and basal ganglia being common sites.
  - Ischaemic strokes (85%) represented by low-density areas (black) within a vascular territory, with loss of grey–white matter differentiation.
  - Mild mass effect may be visualized, e.g. effacement of sulci.
- Colour Doppler ultrasound:
  - Visualizes any stenosis of the internal carotid arteries, along with any changes in blood flow characteristics, allowing evaluation of the need for internal carotid endarterectomy or endovascular stenting.
- Magnetic resonance angiography (MRA):
  - Demonstrates patency of arteries (e.g. stenosis, occlusions, aneurysms and arteriovenous malformations) without the use of contrast media.

- Arteriography:
  - Requires use of contrast material.
  - Less commonly conducted since the use of carotid Dopplers and MRA as it is an invasive test.

Multiple sclerosis

- MRI scan:
  - High signal foci in the periventricular deep white matter on T_2- weighted and FLAIR (fluid-attenuated inversion-recovery sequences).

MICRO-reference

NICE guidelines: Multiple Sclerosis (CG08). Diagnosis and management in primary and secondary care. http://www.nice.org.uk/nicemedia/pdf/cg008guidance.pdf (accessed 05/01/11).

Spinal cord pathology

- Plain radiograph:
  - Allows visualization of the alignment of the spine.
  - May show disc space narrowing, osteophyte formation, and spondylolithesis.
- MRI:
  - Investigation of choice to diagnose degenerative disc disease.
  - Allows visualization of bony canal narrowing and of the spinal theca.
  - Gold standard in the assessment of cord compression.
  - Allows diagnosis of spinal cord tumours by detecting expansion of the cord, reduction of CSF and focal masses which are often cystic.
- CT scan:
  - Allow visualization of bony canal narrowing and of the spinal theca.
- Myelography:
  - Rarely conducted since the introduction of MRI scans.
  - Involves the injection of contrast into the spinal theca via a lumbar puncture, allowing visualization of the spinal cord and nerve roots.

MISCELLANEOUS INVESTIGATIONS

This section will aim to give a brief overview of miscellaneous investigations that may be conducted within the management of patients under the care of neurology.

Neurophysiological tests
- EEG (electroencephalography):
  - Scalp electrodes used to measure electrical impulses of the brain matter below the electrode, which is compared to neighbouring electrodes acting as points of reference.
  - Often conducted simultaneously with video telemetry, with seizures being diagnosed only when the EEG is on the patient during the seizure, while being witnessed/filmed, to avoid false negative or false positive interpretations.
  - Flashing lights can be employed to precipitate seizure activity.
  - Invaluable in diagnosing epilepsy and classifying seizures, but also used in diagnosing encephalitis, comas, Creutzfeldt–Jakob disease (CJD) and subacute sclerosing panencephalitis.
  - Records rhythmic activities which are interpreted by specialists. Some common rhythms include:
    - 3 per second spike and wave which are symmetrical and bilateral: absence seizures and other primary generalized epilepsy syndrome;
    - focal slow wave activity: underlying structural lesion;
    - periodic complexes: CJD.
- Electromyography (EMG):
  - A concentric needle electrode is inserted into voluntary muscle, with amplified recording being viewed on an oscilloscope and heard through a speaker.
  - Records spontaneous and voluntary electrical activity of muscle.
- Nerve conduction studies:
  - Aids diagnosis of neuropathies and nerve entrapments by assessing the transmission of impulses along an individual nerve of interest.
  - Nerve stimulated electrically via a surface electrode, while simultaneously recording sensory and motor action potentials along the nerve by other surface electrodes.
  - The amplitude of response, the latency to the beginning of the response and the conduction velocity are measured.
  - A reduced conduction velocity indicates demyelination, a reduced amplitude suggests axonal loss.
- Evoked potentials:
  - Uses EEG electrodes to record central responses (at the optical cortex) to peripheral stimuli.
  - Visually evoked responses (VERs): speed of response delayed in patients with optic neuritis (regardless of visual loss), aiding the diagnosis of multiple sclerosis.
  - Brainstem auditory evoked responses: uses sound as a stimulus to allow neurosurgical assessment of brain

- Somatosensory potentials: uses sensory stimulus at a limb to allow neurosurgical assessment of spinal cord.

Temporal artery biopsy

- This is used in the diagnosis of giant cell arteritis, requiring a minimum of 1 centimetre as the disease process may be patchy.

MICRO-print

Other possible neurological tests

- Goldmann or Humphrey visual perimetry
  - Used to assess patients' visual fields, investigating for any scotomas.
  - Goldmann perimetry is more sensitive in assessing the peripheral vision and the ability to perceive moving targets.
  - Humphrey fields are useful to assess central fields and the ability to perceive static targets.
  - Commonly used to assess the visual fields of patients with idiopathic intracranial hypertension.
- Tensilon test (edrophonium test)
  - Used as a diagnostic test in myasthenia gravis.
  - Involves the injection of a fast-acting anti-acetylcholinesterase (prevents the breakdown of acetylcholine), which competitively competes with acetylcholine receptor antibodies.
  - When given intravenously (with atropine to prevent cardiovascular side effects), fatigability improves in seconds, lasting for 2–3 minutes, indicating a positive test.

---

11 Rheumatology and orthopaedics

11.1 BLOOD TESTS

- Full blood count (FBC):
    - Anaemia may be due to chronic inflammatory disease, such as rheumatoid arthritis (RA), or from chronic blood loss associated with non-steroidal anti-inflammatory drug (NSAID) use.
    - Infections may lead to neutrophilia, but this may also be a sign of long-term steroid use or inflammatory diseases.
    - Suppressed bone marrow as a result of disease-modifying anti-rheumatic drugs (DMARDs) or diseases such as systemic lupus erythematosus (SLE) can lead to leucopenia.
    - Reactive thrombocytosis may occur secondary to active inflammatory disease, infection or malignancy.
- Urea and electrolytes (U + E):
    - Gout is a recognized cause of nephropathy due to urate deposition in the kidneys, so assessing the estimated glomerular filtration rate (eGFR) may be helpful.
    - Hypovolaemia as a result of orthopaedic fractures and surgery may result in pre-renal failure, so daily U + Es are conducted post-operatively to monitor the trends in urea and creatinine levels.
    - NSAID use for inflammatory diseases can contribute towards the development of renal failure.
- Calcium levels:
    - Hypercalcaemia may be due to diseases such as bony metastases and primary or tertiary hyperparathyroidism.
    - Hypocalcaemia may be due to diseases such as osteomalacia and rickets.
- Parathyroid hormone (PTH) levels:
    - In primary hyperparathyroidism, PTH is generally raised, and is likely to be from a parathyroid adenoma, which can lead to hypercalcaemia and raised alkaline phosphatase (ALP).
    - A normal PTH level in patients with hypercalcaemia indicates an error in the negative feedback loop.

- Vitamin D levels:
  - These are often low in osteomalacia and rickets (the exception being vitamin D-resistant rickets).
- Liver function tests (LFTs):
  - Low albumin levels correlate directly with disease severity in patients with rheumatoid arthritis.
  - Some drugs such as NSAIDs can be hepatotoxic and so assessing liver function is important.
  - Liver disease, Paget's disease, osteomalacia, primary sclerosing cholangitis, bony metastases and polyarteritis nodosa can all lead to increased ALP.
- Clotting screen:
  - Clotting or bleeding disorders, such as haemophilia, sickle cell disease or von Willebrand's disease (rarely), can cause haemarthrosis of a joint.
  - A routine clotting screen is performed before surgery to identify any coagulopathies.
- Blood cultures:
  - Infective organisms may be identified by culturing blood withdrawn prior to antibiotic treatment, e.g. in osteomyelitis.
- Erythrocyte sedimentation rate (ESR):
  - Raised ESR levels are found in polymyalgia rheumatica, osteomyelitis, temporal arteritis, psoriatic arthritis, ankylosing spondylitis, reactive arthritis and rheumatoid arthritis.

MICRO-print

Although hyperuricaemia increases the risk of gout, note that gout can occur with normal uric acid levels (but rarely in the lower half of the normal range). Asymptomatic hyperuricaemia is far more common than gout.

- C-reactive protein (CRP):
  - This may be raised in reactive arthritis and rheumatoid arthritis, and also in acute infection.
- Uric acid:
  - Prolonged hyperuricaemia increases the risk of gout.
- Creatine kinase (CK):
  - CK-MM may be due to myositis or other skeletal muscle damage, e.g. rhabdomyolysis.
- Autoantibodies:
  The main autoantibodies associated with rheumatological disease are as follows.
  - **Antinuclear antibodies** (ANAs) are antibodies to nuclear antigens.

- Positive ANA simply indicates that the patient's blood contains antibodies to the nuclei of the sample cells used in the test. The ANAs specific to their antigens are:
  - **anti-double stranded DNA** (anti-dsDNA) very specific to SLE;
  - **anti-Smith** (anti-Sm) associated with SLE (especially renal lupus);
  - **rheumatoid factor** (RF) associated with rheumatoid arthritis;
  - **anti-centromere** associated with limited cutaneous scleroderma (CREST syndrome) in 70% of patients: highly specific;
  - **anti-Ro** (SS-A) associated with Sjögren's syndrome;
  - **anti-La** (SS-B) associated with Sjögren's syndrome;
  - **anti-topoisomerase II** (anti-SCL-70) associated with diffuse cutaneous scleroderma (in 30% of patients);
  - **anti-ribonucleoprotein (anti-RNP)** associated with mixed connective tissue disease.
- **Anti-cyclic citrullinated peptide** (anti-CCP) is highly specific for rheumatoid arthritis and may be detected years prior to disease onset.
- **Anti-neutrophil cytoplasmic antibodies** (ANCA), of which two main patterns seen:
  - **perinuclear ANCA (pANCA)** associated with microscopic polyangiitis, Churg–Strauss syndrome;
  - **cytoplasmic ANCA (cANCA)** strongly associated with Wegener's granulomatosis and elevated in some cases of microscopic polyangiitis.
- **Anti-Jo-1** is associated with dermatomyositis and polymyositis.
- **Antiphospholipid antibodies (APAs)** are found in antiphospholipid syndrome, where they are associated with venous and arterial thrombosis. They include:
  - anticardiolipin antibody;
  - lupus anticoagulase antibody.

11.2 SYNOVIAL FLUID ANALYSIS

SYNOVIAL FLUID COLLECTION

- Indications:
  - Diagnostic indications
    - unexplained arthritis with synovial effusion;
    - suggestion of an infected joint;
    - suspicion of crystal-induced arthritis;
    - evaluation of therapeutic response in septic arthritis.
  - Therapeutic indications:
    - drainage of septic joint;
      relief of elevated intra-articular pressure;

     – injection of medications, e.g. steroids;

     – evacuation of a painful haemarthrosis.

- Contraindications:
  - Severe coagulopathy.
  - Severe thrombocytopenia.
  - Overlying cellulitis.
- Complications:
  - Iatrogenic infection: the risk of inducing joint infection is low when a sterile technique is used.
  - Tendon injury, rupture, nerve and blood vessel injury, which can result from improper needle insertion – very rare.

MICRO-facts

Synovial fluid aspirations are the most important investigation in suspected septic or crystal arthropathy. It involves the aspiration of synovial fluid from the joint space, possible from most peripheral joints. This is conducted as an aseptic technique, with or without the aid of ultrasound guidance.

MACROSCOPIC APPEARANCE OF SYNOVIAL FLUID

- Note that the macroscopic appearances of aspirates are **indicative and not diagnostic**.
- For example, a septic joint aspirate may not always reveal a cloudy aspirate and so a clear sample from an acutely swollen joint should still be sent for Gram staining and microscopy.

Table 11.1 Synovial fluid analysis.

APPEARANCE OF THE SYNOVIAL FLUID	SIGNIFICANCE
Clear or slightly yellow (not purulent)	Normal
Cloudy	Indicates increased cell count possibly due to inflammation or septic arthritis
Frank pus	Indicates septic arthritis; but can occasionally occur in crystal arthropathies
Blood stained	Can indicate haemarthrosis; however, this may also be a result of blood vessel puncture whilst aspirating

GRAM STAIN AND CULTURE OF SYNOVIAL FLUID

- Synovial fluid Gram stain and culture should always be performed to exclude infection of a symptomatic joint.
- The aspirate should also be routinely sent for polarized light microscopy as crystal arthropathy is a key differential for septic arthritis.
- The commonest organisms are *Staphylococcus aureus* and streptococci, with *Haemophilus influenzae* type b only significantly affecting the 7–36 month group.
- Suspect gonococcus in young sexually active adults.

POLARIZED LIGHT MICROSCOPY OF THE SYNOVIAL FLUID

> **MICRO-facts**
>
> The sooner the synovial fluid is analysed under polarized light, the higher the chance of seeing crystals.

- Aspirated fluid should be sent for polarized light microscopy if **a crystal-induced disease** (e.g. gout or pseudogout) is suspected, e.g. in a joint with acute erythema, pain and swelling in the first metatarsophalangeal joint, mid-foot or ankle.
- **Types of crystals** that may be found in joint aspirations include:
  - monosodium urate crystals:
    - needle-shaped;
    - strongly negatively birefringent – crystals parallel to the plane of light appear yellow, and crystals at right angles appear blue;
    - intra- or extracellular crystals;
    - seen in gout.
  - Calcium pyrophosphate dihydrate (CPPD) crystals:
    - either rhomboid or rod-shaped;
    - weakly positively birefringent;
    - intra- or extracellular crystals;
    - seen in calcium pyrophosphate dihydrate disease, also known as 'pseudogout'.
  - Basic calcium phosphate (BCP) crystals:
    - found in severe rheumatic conditions such as osteoarthritis (60% of cases);
    - definitive assay for BCP crystals in synovial fluid is not readily available;
    - clumped crystals can be identified only with transmission electron microscopy;
    - the clumps are not birefringent under polarized light.
  - Calcium oxalate crystals:
    - crystals are positively birefringent and bipyramidal in shape;
    - found in calcium oxalate arthritis (rare);

- radiography and laboratory tests are not diagnostic, but the treatment is the same as for CPPD disease.
- Material aspirated from tophi can be examined in the same way.
- Note that the absence of crystals does not rule out the diagnosis.

11.3 OTHER COMMON RHEUMATOLOGY AND ORTHOPAEDICS INVESTIGATIONS

SWABS AND CULTURES

- Wound swabs and throat swabs may be positive and indicate a source of infection for septic joints.
- Urine microscopy and culture may also reveal a source for joint sepsis.

RADIOLOGY

For more information, please refer to Chapter 5, Radiology.

Osteoporosis
- Plain radiographs:
  - These require significantly reduced bone mass (osteopenia) to be detected on plain films, especially of the spine. They are not very sensitive.
  - Commonly presenting as skeletal fractures as a result of minor trauma and vertebral fractures, including vertebral compression fractures.
- Bone densitometry scans:
  - Dual-energy X-ray absorption (DEXA) scan
    - T score compares the patient's bone mineral density values with those of young normal patients;
    - Z score compares the patient's bone mineral density values with those of an age-matched normal patient;
    - bone mineral density T score of 2.5 standard deviations below the mean or lower is diagnostic of osteoporosis;
    - bone mineral density T score of 1.0–2.4 standard deviations below the mean is diagnostic of osteopenia;
    - bone mineral density T score of 1 standard deviation below the mean and above is within the normal range.

Osteoarthritis
- Plain radiograph:
  - Most weight-bearing joints can be affected, especially knees, spine, hips and shoulders and hands.

MICRO-facts

Features of osteoarthritis include:

- osteophyte formation at joint margins;
- non-uniform joint space narrowing;
- subchondral cysts;
- subchondral sclerosis.

Rheumatoid arthritis

- Ultrasound:
  - Can detect synovitis at an early stage.
  - Slowly replacing the need for plain radiographs.
- Plain radiographs:
  - Symmetrical distribution, most commonly affecting synovial joints, especially the small joints of the hands and feet.
  - Often repeated after several months in patients who have persistent symptoms, but normal initial radiographs.

MICRO-facts

Features to look for in rheumatoid arthritis that can be seen on plain radiographs tend to be seen first in the joints of the hands and feet:

- initially joint space widening, followed by uniform joint space narrowing;
- marginal erosions, eventually spreading across articular surface;
- periarticular osteoporosis;
- soft-tissue swelling.

- Computed tomography (CT) scans or magnetic resonance imaging (MRI) scans:
  - For severe disease, giving detailed extensive imaging of a joint.
  - Can detect erosions sooner that on radiographs.

Crystal arthropathies

- Plain radiographs:
  - In acute attacks, soft tissue swelling will be evident.
  - Chronic changes include:
    - joint effusions and swellings;
    - erosions appearing as 'punched out' lesions, lying away from the articular surfaces;
    - tophus formation in soft tissues, around joints.

Clinical specialties

Ankylosing spondylitis

- Plain films:
  - Spinal changes, creating a 'bamboo spine' image, include:
    - squaring of the vertebrae;
    - paraspinal ligamentous calcification;
    - syndesmophyte formation.
  - Sacroiliac joints showing:
    - blurring and poor definition of joint margins;
    - erosions and sclerosis, completing joint fusion.
  - peripheral joints:
    - erosive arthropathy may be seen.

Rickets

- Plain radiographs:
  - Generalized reduced bone density.
  - Widening of growth plates and epiphysis.
  - Fraying of the metaphysis giving a cupped edge appearance.
  - Bowing and curving of the long bones.
  - 'Rickety rosary' of the anterior ribs due to bullous enlargement.

Osteomyelitis

- Plain radiographs:
  - Conventional radiography should always be the first imaging modality, as it provides an overview of the anatomy and the pathologic conditions of the bone and soft tissues of the region of interest.
  - Initially show soft-tissue swelling, and blurring of the soft tissue planes. In pyogenic infections, the first change in bone indicates that the infection has been present for 2–3 weeks. On occasion gas is present in the soft tissues. If initially normal, films repeated in 2 weeks.
  - Typical early bony changes include: periosteal thickening, lytic lesions, endosteal scalloping, osteopenia, loss of trabecular architecture, and new bone apposition.
- Ultrasound:
  - Most useful in the diagnosis of fluid collections, periosteal involvement, and surrounding soft tissue abnormalities and may provide guidance for diagnostic or therapeutic aspiration, drainage, or tissue biopsy.
- Isotope bone scans:
  - Will highlight increased bone activity in affected joints.
- CT scans and MRI scans:
  - Sensitive in detecting infection and displaying any soft tissue changes.

Paget's disease

- Plain radiographs:
  - Skull, spine, pelvis and long bones are frequently imaged, but any bone may be involved.

- May include:
  - bone expansion, e.g. increased size of diploe of the skull enlargement of pubis and ischium, and widening of long bones;
  - generalized sclerosis with trabecular thickening;
  - diploic thickening producing a 'cotton wool' appearance of skull in the chronic phase.
- Isotope tests:
  - May show increased isotope uptake in affected bones.

Bone tumours
- Plain radiographs:
  - May show area of bone destruction and loss of bone architecture.
- CT and MRI:
  - Allows evaluation of tumour.
  - Allows assessment of the involvement of surrounding structures and metastatic spread.

Fractures
- Plain radiographs:
  - May show the fracture line and associated soft-tissue swelling.
- CT scans:
  - Highly sensitive in detecting fractures and associated surrounding damage, especially with viewing techniques such as 'bone windows'.
  - Used when a high clinical suspicion remains despite normal plain radiographs or for the pre-surgical assessment of complex fractures.

MICRO-reference

WHO Scientific Group on the Prevention and Management of Osteoporosis, Geneva, Switzerland (2003). Prevention and management of osteoporosis: report of a WHO scientific group. http://whqlibdoc. who.int/trs/who_trs_921.pdf (accessed 1/10/2011).

MICRO-print
Further specific radiology

- Arthrography
  - Involves injection of contrast and air into a joint, especially hips, shoulders and wrist.
  - May include the visualization of contrast under CT, MRI or fluoroscopy.

continued...

continued...

- Ideal for identifying loose bodies or anatomical abnormalities, such as labral tears.
- Bone scintigraphy (isotope bone scanning)
  - Shows an outline of the body with areas highlighted where the isotope has accumulated.
  - Sensitive in identifying the presence of active disease, not specific in identifying which disease.
  - Increased uptake can identify sites of fractures, arthritis, infection, neoplasm and Paget's disease.
  - Decreased uptake can occur in some neoplasms and avascular bone.
- Quantitative CT scan
  - Less accurate, more expensive and requires higher radiation doses than other bone density measurements.

Table 11.2 Types of fracture.

TYPE OF FRACTURE	DESCRIPTION
Comminuted	A fracture resulting in many pieces
Impacted	Due to fracture fragments being compressed together, appearing as a sclerotic line from bone overlap
Stress	Results from repeated or pressured injury
Pathological	Fractures occurring in diseased bones after minor injury, e.g. bone tumours, Paget's disease and osteoporosis
Greenstick	Bending of a long bone with a break of the cortex on the other side
Epiphyseal	Occur at the epiphyseal plates in children – classified using Salter–Harris classification
Avulsion	As a result of a tendon or ligament pulling a fragment of bone off its insertion, usually in children or adolescents
Compound	A fracture resulting in an open wound, i.e. with bone protruding through skin

MISCELLANEOUS INVESTIGATIONS

- Biopsies:
  - Note that some pathologies, such as myositis, may be patchy and biopsy may miss the affected part of the organ, giving a falsely negative biopsy result.

Table 11.3 Biopsies performed in rheumatological investigation.

BIOPSY LOCATION	EXAMPLES OF PATHOLOGIES SUSPECTED
Muscle	Myositis
Blood vessels	Vasculitis
Nerve	Vasculitis
Skin	Vasculitis
Kidney	Connective tissue disease involving kidney
Bone	Primary bone tumour, osteomalacia and renal osteodystrophy

- Schirmer tear test:
  - This is used in diagnosis of Sjögren's syndrome and keratoconjunctivitis sicca (dry eyes).
  - A standard strip of filter paper placed on the inside of the lower eyelid.
  - Wetting of the paper by < 10 mm in 5 minutes indicates defective tear production.
- EMG and nerve conduction:
  - These are used in the diagnosis of neuromuscular problems, distinguishing between muscular disease and neuropathic disorders.
  - In myositis, there is a typical triad of changes in EMG:
    i. spontaneous fibrillation potentials at rest;
    ii. polyphasic or short-duration potentials on voluntary contraction;
    iii. repetitive potentials on mechanical stimulation of the nerve.

MICRO-print
See Chapter 10, Neurology, for further details on EMG and nerve conduction studies.

- Arthroscopy:
  - Allows direct visualization of a joint.
  - For example, in osteoarthritis, fissuring and surface erosion of the cartilage may be seen.
  - Often used as a diagnostic investigation, however surgical treatment may also be given via arthroscopy under strict criteria such as when there is a clear history of mechanical locking allowing effective arthroscopy treatment (e.g. repairing or trimming meniscal tears, or removing loose bodies).
  - Often conducted on the shoulder or knee joints, but may also be conducted on the ankle and hip joints.

Clinical specialties

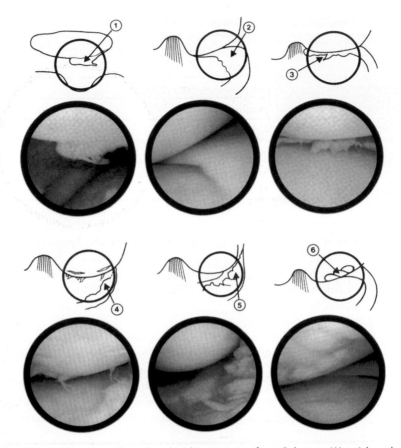

Fig. 11.1 Arthroscopy. Reproduced with permission from Solomon, Warwick and Nayagam, *Apley's system of orthopaedics and fractures*, 9th edn. Fig. 20.12.

Part III

Self-assessment

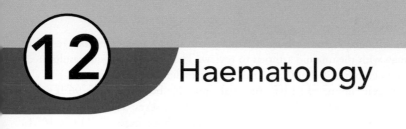

Haematology

Questions

HAEMATOLOGICAL DIAGNOSES: EMQs

For each of the following clinical scenarios, please choose the correct diagnosis. Each option may be used once, more than once or not at all.

Diagnostic options

1) Bacterial infection
2) Lymphocytopenia
3) Macrocytic anaemia
4) Microcytic hyperchromic anaemia
5) Microcytic hypochromic anaemia
6) Neutropenia
7) Normocytic anaemia
8) Thrombocytopenia
9) Thrombocytosis
10) Viral infection

Question 1:

You are a trainee doctor working in primary care when a young 20-year-old woman comes to see you complaining of tiredness and lethargy. You take a full history and find that she also complains of heavy periods. You decide to perform a full blood count. What are you expecting this to show?

Question 2:

You are the junior doctor on the gastroenterology team and have been asked to clerk in a confused 60-year-old woman. Her daughter tells you that her mother has recently been diagnosed with dementia and that when her GP performed some routine tests an abnormality was found and so she was sent to you because of her history of a partial gastrectomy. Her daughter reports that she has been forgetting to attend her healthcare appointments recently. You have a suspicion as to what the abnormality might be and so take some blood and send the samples to the laboratory. What abnormality are you looking for?

Question 3:

You are a trainee doctor working in primary care and are given the blood results of a woman with rheumatoid arthritis to review. The full blood count results are:

Haemoglobin of 9.1 g/dL (normal range for females: 11.5–16 g/dL)
Mean cell volume of 81.0 fL (normal range for both sexes: 76–96 fL)
Platelets of 394×10^9/L (normal range for both sexes: 150–400×10^9/L)
White cell count of 9.0×10^9/L (normal range for both sexes: 4.0–11.0×10^9/L)

What do these results show?

Diagnostic options

1) Bacterial infection
2) Lymphocytopenia
3) Macrocytic anaemia
4) Microcytic hyperchromic anaemia
5) Microcytic hypochromic anaemia

6) Neutropenia
7) Normocytic anaemia
8) Thrombocytopenia
9) Thrombocytosis
10) Viral infection

Question 4:

You are the junior doctor on-call and have been asked to see an elderly 79-year-old man who is a little short of breath and is coughing up green sputum. The nurse has completed her observations and he has a respiratory rate of 20 breaths per minute and a temperature of 38.4°C. You send away for a full blood count and the results return as:

Haemoglobin of 15.3 g/dL (normal range for males: 13.5–18 g/dL)
Mean cell volume of 81.0 fL (normal range for both sexes: 76–96 fL)
Platelets of 394×10^9/L (normal range for both sexes: 150–400×10^9/L)
White cell count of 17.1×10^9/L (normal range for both sexes: 4.0–11.0×10^9/L)
Neutrophils: 13.9×10^9/L (normal range for both sexes: 2.0–7.5×10^9/L)
Lymphocytes 3.0×10^9/L (normal range for both sexes: 1.5–4.0×10^9/L)

What do these results show?

Question 5:

You are the junior doctor on-call and have been asked to see a 40-year-old female patient who has been admitted by an endocrinology consultant from clinic. This woman was recently started on carbimazole for her hyperthyroidism and was being followed-up in clinic. The consultant was concerned when they saw her recent blood results. These were:

Haemoglobin of 13.4 g/dL (normal range for females: 11.5–16 g/dL)
Mean cell volume of 86.0 fL (normal range for both sexes: 76–96 fL)

Platelets of 370×10^9/L (normal range for both sexes: $150–400 \times 10^9$/L)
White cell count of 3.5×10^9/L (normal range for both sexes: $4.0–11.0 \times 10^9$/L)
Neutrophils: 0.8×10^9/L (normal range for both sexes: $2.0–7.5 \times 10^9$/L)
Lymphocytes 2.0×10^9/L (normal range for both sexes: $1.5–4.0 \times 10^9$/L)

What do they show?

Question 6:

You are the junior doctor working in general surgery. Three days ago a 27-year-old man was brought to the accident and emergency department following a road traffic incident. He underwent emergency splenectomy. You are monitoring his progress and you look at his blood results from today. These are:

Haemoglobin of 13.7 g/dL (normal range for males: $13.5–18$ g/dL)
Mean cell volume of 79.0 fL (normal range for both sexes: $76–96$ fL)
Platelets of 732×10^9/L (normal range for both sexes: $150–400 \times 10^9$/L)
White cell count of 10.1×10^9/L (normal range for both sexes: $4.0–11.0 \times 10^9$/L)
Neutrophils: 7.2×10^9/L (normal range for both sexes: $2.0–7.5 \times 10^9$/L)
Lymphocytes 2.7×10^9/L (normal range for both sexes: $1.5–4.0 \times 10^9$/L)

What do they show?

HAEMATOLOGICAL INVESTIGATIONS: SBA

For the following clinical scenario, please choose the single most appropriate answer from the options below.

Question 7:

You are the junior doctor on the haematology ward and are asked to see a 16-year-old youth who is known to have a significant haematological condition. He has been poorly compliant with this treatment and it has been found that he has had bleeding into some of his joints, which are now painful. You decided to perform a coagulation screen. Which abnormality from the list below would you most expect to find given this young man's disease?
1) Deranged international normalized ratio
2) Prolonged activated partial thromboplastin time
3) Prolonged prothrombin time
4) Reduced von Willebrand's factor
5) Thrombocytopenia

Answers

HAEMATOLOGICAL DIAGNOSES: EMQs

Answer 1:

5) Microcytic hypochromic anaemia: This patient has menorrhagia, a common complaint in young females. This condition often results in iron-deficiency anaemia, which would explain the tiredness and lethargy. In iron-deficiency anaemia the red blood cells appear small (microcytic) and pale (hypochromic).

Answer 2:

3) Macrocytic anaemia: This patient has had a partial gastrectomy, which makes her susceptible to B12 deficiency due to decreased production of intrinsic factor by the stomach. It is likely that B12 replacement therapy would have been commenced and so she should have been having B12 injections every 3 months. Unfortunately, however, her daughter reports that she has been confused and has been missing appointments so she may well have become B12 deficient.

Answer 3:

7) Normocytic anaemia: Patients with rheumatoid arthritis are susceptible to both anaemia of chronic disease (normocytic anaemia) and iron-deficiency anaemia (due to blood loss from peptic ulcers as a consequence of taking non-steroidal anti-inflammatory medication). This patient's results indicate that she is anaemic with a normal mean cell volume, meaning that she has a normocytic anaemia. Her platelets and white cell count are within normal ranges.

Answer 4:

1) Bacterial infection: This man has the signs of a respiratory tract infection (green sputum, shortness of breath and pyrexia). In addition his white cell count is elevated. It is apparent that this man's neutrophils are above the normal range while his lymphocytes are normal, therefore indicating the infective cause to be bacterial.

Answer 5:

6) Neutropenia: This patient's blood results show a low white cell count and a very low neutrophil count (with normal lymphocyte count). A known side effect of carbimazole is neutropenia and, due to all the adverse consequences of having a low white cell count, it is very important that this is managed accordingly.

Answer 6:

9) Thrombocytosis: Splenectomy patients can develop a secondary reactive thrombocytosis in the post-operative period as evidenced by the elevated platelet count in this case. The most important clinical relevance of this fact is that early mobilization is needed due to the increased risk of thrombi from the high platelet concentration.

HAEMATOLOGICAL INVESTIGATIONS: SBA

Answer 7:

2) Prolonged activated partial thromboplastin time: This young male patient has a significant haematological condition that has resulted in bleeding into his joints; the most likely diagnosis is therefore either haemophilia A or B. Haemophilia is due to factor VIII or factor IX deficiency (A and B respectively). If someone is poorly compliant with therapy then they will become factor deficient and therefore a prolonged activated partial thromboplastin time on a clotting screen will be detected. The answer is not reduced von Willebrand's factor as those with haemophilia are not deficient in this factor. Although von Willebrand's disease may cause bleeding, it is usually mild, e.g. mucosal bleeding. Haemarthrosis would therefore be unlikely. The answer is not a prolonged prothrombin time as this is dependent on clotting factors I, II, V, VII and X (i.e. not factor VIII or factor IX). Since an INR is based on the prothrombin time it cannot be this answer either. Finally, the answer is not thrombocytopenia because those with haemophilia are not deficient in platelets, only one of the two clotting factors already mentioned.

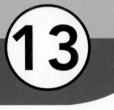

Biochemistry

Questions

DIAGNOSTIC INVESTIGATIONS INTERPRETATION: EMQs

For each of the following clinical scenarios, please choose the correct diagnosis. Each option can be used once, more than once or not at all.

Diagnostic options

1) Acute renal failure
2) Anaemia
3) Chronic renal failure
4) Diuretic therapy
5) Excess 5% dextrose solution
6) Excess 0.9% saline
7) Excessive beta-blockade
8) Hartmann's solution
9) Hyperkalaemia
10) Hypokalaemia

Question 1:

You are the junior doctor on-call and you have been asked to review the blood results of a 92-year-old female inpatient. She has known heart failure and was documented to have pulmonary oedema on admission 6 days ago. This has been aggressively treated. The urea and electrolyte profile is shown below.

Na^+: 127 mmol/L (normal range: 135–145 mmol/L)
K^+: 4.1 mmol/L (normal range: 3.5–5.3 mmol/L)
Urea: 6.6 mmol/L (normal range: 2.5–6.7 mmol)
Creatinine: 83 µmol/L (normal range: 79–118 µmol/L)
Cl^-: 98 mmol/L (normal range: 95–105 mmol/L)
HCO_3^-: 28 mmol/L (normal range: 24–30 mmol/L)

What is the likely cause of these results?

Question 2:

You are the junior doctor on-call and a worried medical student hands you an ECG that she has just performed on a patient. What does it show?

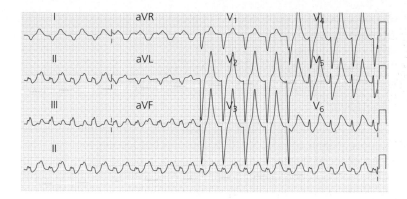

Fig. 13.1 Biochemistry question 2.

Question 3:

You are the junior doctor on-call and have clerked in a 72-year-old man who has had diarrhoea and vomiting for the past 3 days. He has eaten and drunk little during this episode of illness. On examination you find he has reduced skin turgor and dry mucus membranes. You request, among other things, a urea and electrolyte profile, the results are shown below.

Na$^+$: 130 mmol/L (normal range: 135–145 mmol/L)
K$^+$: 6.0 mmol/L (normal range: 3.5–5.0 mmol/L)
Urea: 14.1 mmol/L (normal range: 2.5–6.7 mmol)
Creatinine: 190 μmol/L (normal range: 79–118 μmol/L)
Cl$^-$: 98 mmol/L (normal range: 95–105 mmol/L)
HCO$_3^-$: 28 mmol/L (normal range: 24–30 mmol/L)

What do the results show?

LIVER FUNCTION TEST INTERPRETATION: EMQs

For each of the following clinical scenarios, which all relate to liver function tests, please choose the most accurate answer from the options below. Each option may be used once, more than once or not at all.

Diagnostic options

1) Elevated bilirubin only
2) Elevated gamma-glutamyl transpeptidase (GGT), alkaline phosphatase and bilirubin
3) Elevated transaminases
4) Low alkaline phosphatase only
5) Low alanine aminotransferase (ALT) only

6) Low aspartate transaminase (AST) only
7) Low bilirubin
8) Low transaminases (AST and ALT)
9) Low GGT and alkaline phosphatase
10) Low GGT only

Question 4:

You are the junior doctor on-call and a GP refers a 45-year-old woman to you with upper abdominal pain. She feels nauseous but has not vomited. The pain came on earlier in the day and has continued to progress despite being 'on/off' in nature. On examination she is clearly in pain with tenderness in her right upper quadrant, and is jaundiced. She is afebrile and her white cell count is normal. What would you expect her liver function tests to show?

Question 5:

You are a trainee doctor working in primary care when a 29-year-old woman presents with vague gastrointestinal symptoms with no worrying features. Examination provided no significant findings. Without being overly concerned, you request some simple blood tests to make sure there is nothing sinister underlying these symptoms. On reviewing the results you are surprised to find that the liver function tests are markedly deranged. Concerned, you ask to see her again and on further questioning she reveals that she has recently started a new relationship with a man from Cyprus and has been having unprotected sex with him. What do you think the liver function tests show?

TUMOUR MARKER INTERPRETATION: EMQs

For each of the following clinical scenarios, which all relate to tumour markers, please choose the correct diagnosis. Each option can be used once, more than once or not at all.

Diagnostic options

1) α-Fetoprotein
2) β-Human chorionic gonadotrophin (β-hCG)
3) β-Human chorionic gonadotrophin and α-fetoprotein
4) CA 15-3
5) CA 19-9
6) CA 27-29
7) CA-125
8) Carcinoembryonic antigen (CEA)
9) NMP22
10) Prostate-specific antigen

Question 6:

A 21-year-old man presented 3 months ago with a painless, irregular lump in the scrotum. This was confirmed as a testicular teratoma and he underwent an orchidectomy. He is now being followed-up and as part of this he has regular blood tests. Which tumour marker or markers would clinicians look for?

Question 7:

You are a trainee doctor working in primary care when a 60-year-old man presents to you complaining of unintentional weight loss but no other symptoms. You note that he only drinks moderately (approximately 10 units per week). Examination reveals slight jaundice, but nothing else of note. Concerned, you organize some routine blood tests and find the liver function tests to be deranged. On questioning, he reveals that during the 1960s and 1970s he was in a rock band and lived a 'heavy' lifestyle with lots of alcohol, drugs and unprotected heterosexual sex. He admits to some intravenous drug use. You request hepatitis B and C serology and he is found to be hepatitis C positive. An ultrasound scan is organized and demonstrates a focal liver lesion suspicious for malignancy. In such a case, which tumour marker or markers would you expect to be elevated?

Question 8:

A 52-year-old woman presented 1 year ago with increasing abdominal distension. On an ultrasound scan she was found to have a large ovarian mass which was later diagnosed as malignant. Appropriate surgical and chemotherapy intervention was subsequently initiated. As part of follow-up, a tumour marker or markers specific to this malignancy are measured. What marker or markers are these?

Answers

DIAGNOSTIC INVESTIGATIONS INTERPRETATION: EMQs

Answer 1:

4) Diuretic therapy: This woman has been aggressively treated for pulmonary oedema and therefore it is highly likely that the hyponatraemia is a result of diuretic therapy. Her urea is at the upper end of the normal range and this is probably due to her age. Nonetheless you would want to monitor this to ensure that she does not progress into renal failure. Frail elderly people (women in particular) frequently have low creatinine due to their reduced muscle mass, and so a high creatinine may still be in the 'normal' range but be high for them. Estimated glomerular filtration rate gives a more accurate measurement of renal function (see Chapter 2, Clinical chemistry).

Answer 2:

9) Hyperkalaemia: This ECG is classical of hyperkalaemia, it has flattened P waves, a broad QRS complex, a 'sine wave' pattern, and tall-tented T waves. The medical student is right to be concerned: if this is not corrected then the patient may develop a fatal arrhythmia.

Answer 3:

1) Acute renal failure: This patient is acutely dehydrated (as evidenced by the history and physical examination) and his blood results show that he has a high urea and creatinine. In addition his potassium is high as a consequence of his poor renal function (normally the kidneys excrete potassium). Hypovolaemia is a common cause of pre-renal failure and this must be treated quickly in order to prevent the onset of acute tubular necrosis. An answer of 'chronic renal failure' is incorrect as there is no mention of his past medical history and in the clinical context of gastroenteritis, acute renal failure is more likely.

LIVER FUNCTION TEST INTERPRETATION: EMQs

Answer 4:

2) Elevated gamma-glutamyl transpeptidase (GGT), alkaline phosphatase and bilirubin: This patient has a history and examination suggestive of choledocholithiasis – a gallstone blocking the common bile duct, causing an 'obstructive' liver function test pattern. This means that the GGT and alkaline phosphatase are markedly raised with the transaminases (ALT and AST) either normal or marginally elevated. The obstruction also results in an elevated bilirubin as bile is unable to pass from the liver to the duodenum via the common bile duct.

Answer 5:

3) Elevated transaminases: This patient's history puts her at risk of viral hepatitis (e.g. hepatitis B or hepatitis C). In hepatitis, the liver is inflamed and the damaged hepatocytes release transaminases (AST and ALT respectively) into the blood stream. As this is a liver problem and not an outflow tract problem you would expect to see a 'hepatitic' pattern in the liver function tests: raised transaminases (AST and ALT) with normal or marginally elevated GGT and alkaline phosphatase.

TUMOUR MARKER INTERPRETATION: EMQs

Answer 6:

3) β-Human chorionic gonadotrophin and α-fetoprotein: Testicular cancers are most commonly germ cell tumours and in the 20- to 30-year-old age group they are most commonly teratomas. Germ cell tumours (particularly teratomas) cause elevated levels of β-human chorionic gonadotrophin and α-fetoprotein and can be monitored to detect recurrence.

Answer 7:

1) α-Fetoprotein: As well as being elevated in germ cell tumours, it is also raised substantially in hepatocellular carcinoma. Having hepatitis C puts this patient at significant risk of developing this cancer (as indeed this man's history would suggest) This case should highlight the need for taking a comprehensive history, particularly if presented with an unusual case.

Answer 8:

7) CA-125: In ovarian malignancies CA-125 is often raised and so is useful for monitoring tumour recurrence.

Questions

For the following clinical scenarios, please choose the single most appropriate answer from the options given.

Question 1:

You are a trainee doctor working in primary care when a 40-year-old woman presents with symptoms suggestive of hyperthyroidism. Initially you suspect that this may be primary hyperthyroidism and send off a blood sample requesting thyroid function status. To your surprise the result suggests secondary hyperthyroidism. What pattern of results would you expect to see?

1) Low T_3/T_4 with low thyroid-stimulating hormone
2) Low T_3/T_4 with raised thyroid-stimulating hormone
3) Normal T_3/T_4 with raised thyroid-stimulating hormone
4) Raised T_3/T_4 with raised thyroid-stimulating hormone
5) Raised T_3/T_4 with low thyroid-stimulating hormone

Question 2:

You are a trainee doctor working in primary care when a 60-year-old man presents complaining of increased weight. He comments that his mood has also changed and that he is feeling depressed. On examination, you notice that he has central obesity and prominent abdominal striae. You also notice a round face. While at your consultation, he repeatedly coughs and mentions that this is non-productive. He is a heavy-smoker. Concerned, you send him for a plain chest radiograph. The reporting radiologist makes a provisional diagnosis of bronchial carcinoma. Given this, you suspect a particular diagnosis regarding the original presenting symptoms and signs. What test, from the list below, could be used to test for this?

1) Blood glucose
2) Dexamethasone suppression test
3) Oral glucose tolerance test
4) Synacthen® test
5) Thyroid function test

Question 3:

You are a trainee doctor working in primary care when a young woman presents to your surgery complaining of vague abdominal pain and fatigue. You are somewhat mystified, but on examination you notice that her skin appears to have darkened. She says she has not been on holiday for over a year and that you are not the first to comment on this. You notice dark palmar creases. Suspecting a diagnosis, you request an investigation to confirm your suspicions. From the list below, which is the most appropriate option?

1) Blood glucose
2) Dexamethasone suppression test
3) Oral glucose tolerance test
4) Synacthen® test
5) Thyroid function test

Question 4:

You are a trainee doctor working in primary care when a young woman presents to your surgery complaining of irregular periods, nipple discharge and visual disturbances. On examination you note the discharge and a bitemporal hemianopia on visual field examination. From the list below, which is the most appropriate investigation?

1) Adrenocorticotrophic hormone (ACTH)
2) Adrenaline
3) Corticotrophin-releasing hormone (CRH)
4) Dopamine
5) Prolactin

Question 5:

You are a trainee doctor working in primary care when a new patient, a 55-year-old man, presents for a diabetic review. He developed diabetes mellitus type 2 when he was 40 years old. While taking the history you note that he has a prominent jaw, large hands, and that his wedding ring appears tight. On questioning he comments that initially the wedding ring fitted well, but over the years it has become increasingly tight. He has had it resized twice. Suspecting that there may be an underlying diagnosis, which investigation from the list below would you like to request?

1) ACTH
2) Adrenaline
3) CRH
4) Insulin-like growth factor-1
5) Prolactin

Question 6:

You are a trainee doctor working in primary care when a 63-year-old obese woman presents to you complaining of vaginal thrush. You are suspicious as this is the fourth time in 2 months she has had the condition. You take a history and she reveals that she has been thirstier of late and that she has been going to the toilet more often. You suspect the two problems might be linked and decide to request an investigation. From the list below, which is the most appropriate?

1) ACTH
2) CRH
3) Growth hormone
4) Oral glucose tolerance test
5) Prolactin

Answers

Answer 1:

4) Raised T$_3$/T$_4$ with raised thyroid-stimulating hormone: Secondary hyperthyroidism occurs as a consequence of excess thyroid-stimulating hormone being produced, e.g. by a pituitary tumour. This results in inappropriately high levels of thyroid-stimulating hormone being secreted, as the tumour doesn't respond to negative feedback. T$_3$/T$_4$ will be high as a consequence of the excess thyroid-stimulating hormone. Secondary hyperthyroidism is uncommon.

Answer 2:

2) Dexamethasone suppression test: The presenting symptoms and signs are suggestive of Cushing's syndrome (central obesity, abdominal striae, moon face and lethargy). Small cell lung cancer may produce ectopic ACTH, and hence lead to Cushing's syndrome. Dexamethasone suppression tests involve giving exogenous dexamethasone. In 'normal' people giving dexamethasone will suppress circulating levels of cortisol, while in those with Cushing's syndrome there will be little suppression. Thyroid function tests are used to assess thyroid status; Synacthen® for hypoadrenalism; blood glucose for diabetes; insulin tolerance test for acromegaly. See Chapter 3, Endocrinology, for more details.

Answer 3:

4) Synacthen® test: The presenting symptoms and signs are suggestive of Addison's disease. Addison's disease results in hypoadrenalism and so the Synacthen test is the most appropriate investigation. In hypoadrenalism you would expect a non-significant rise in cortisol after administration of Synacthen (a synthetic ACTH analogue).

Answer 4:

5) Prolactin: This patient's signs and symptoms are suggestive of high levels of prolactin (glacatorrhoea and oligomenorrhoea) with compression of the optic chiasm (bitemporal hemianopia). A potential cause of this is a prolactin-secreting macroadenoma.

Answer 5:

4) Insulin-like growth factor-1: This patient's signs and symptoms are suggestive of acromegaly (prominent jaw and large hands). Diabetes mellitus is known to be associated with this condition as the excess growth hormone acts against normal insulin production. Insulin-like growth factor-1 is responsible for the soft tissue and skeletal growth (hence the prominent jaw and large hands) and so can be used as a screening test for this condition (growth hormone stimulates insulin-like growth factor-1). The definitive test for acromegaly is the oral glucose tolerance test: glucose inhibits growth hormone production.

Answer 6:

4) Oral glucose tolerance test: This patient is a 63-year-old obese woman, a likely candidate for developing type 2 diabetes. She is complaining of polyuria and polydipsia, which are classical symptoms. In addition she is having multiple episodes of vaginal candidiasis, which is a known complication of having high levels of glucose in the urine. Normally diabetes is diagnosed by blood glucose levels, but if the results are equivocal then an oral glucose tolerance test is performed. From the list this is the only appropriate investigation.

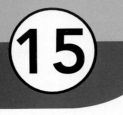

Radiology

Questions

PLAIN RADIOGRAPH INTERPRETATION: EMQs

For each of the following clinical scenarios, all of which focus on radiological investigations, please choose the most likely diagnosis. Each option may be used once, more than once or not at all.

Diagnostic options

1) Bilateral pleural effusion
2) Congestive cardiac failure
3) Left lung mass
4) Left apical pneumothorax
5) Pneumoperitoneum
6) Pulmonary fibrosis
7) Right lower lobe collapse
8) Right apical pneumothorax
9) Right upper lobe collapse
10) Right upper lobe consolidation

Question 1:

What is the diagnosis?

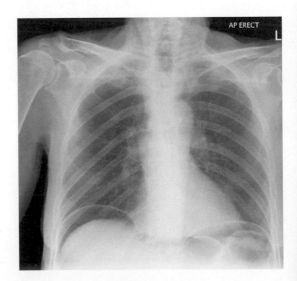

Fig. 15.1 Radiology
question 1.

Question 2:

What is the diagnosis?

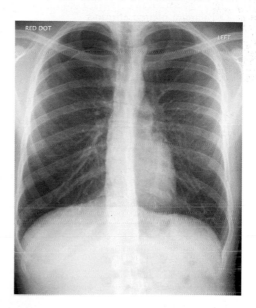

Fig. 15.2 Radiology question 2.

Question 3:

What is the diagnosis?

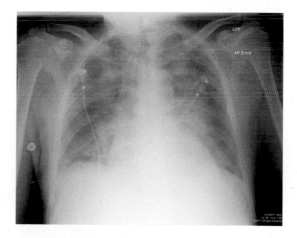

Fig. 15.3 Radiology
question 3.

For each of the following clinical scenarios, all of which focus on radiological investigations, please choose the most likely diagnosis. Each option may be used once, more than once or not at all.

Diagnostic options

1) Bilateral pleural effusion
2) Congestive cardiac failure
3) Left apical pneumothorax
4) Left lower lobe collapse
5) Left lung mass

6) Left upper lobe consolidation
7) Pneumoperitoneum
8) Right apical pneumothorax
9) Right upper lobe collapse
10) Right upper lobe consolidation

Question 4:

What is the diagnosis?

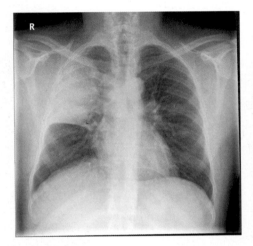

Fig. 15.4 Radiology question 4.

Question 5:

What is the diagnosis?

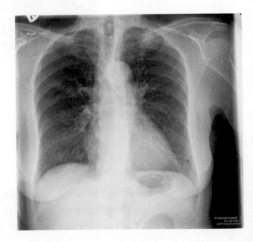

Fig. 15.5 Radiology question 5.

Diagnostic options

1) Bladder malignancy
2) Calculi
3) Inflammatory bowel disease
4) Large bowel obstruction
5) Pneumoperitoneum

6) Polycystic kidneys
7) Renal transplant
8) Small bowel obstruction
9) Toxic megacolon
10) Ureteric malignancy

Question 6:

What is the diagnosis?

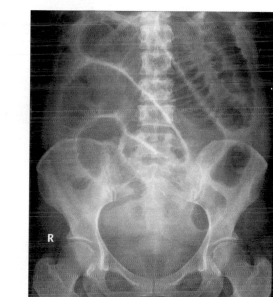

Fig. 15.6 Radiology question 6.

Question 7:
What is the diagnosis?

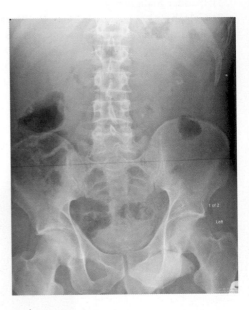

Fig. 15.7 Radiology question 7.

Question 8:
What is the diagnosis?

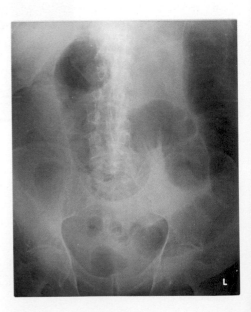

Fig. 15.8 Radiology question 8.

Answers

PLAIN RADIOGAPH INTERPETATION: EMQs

Answer 1:

5) **Pneumoperitoneum:** Gas is seen bilaterally below the hemi-diaphragms. The gas in the peritoneum rises upwards on an erect radiograph, causing it to accumulate below the diaphragm. Note that free gas in the peritoneum usually indicates a visceral perforation. In this radiograph, the lung fields are translucent with no visible masses, and the lung markings are symmetrical throughout the lungs, indicating no lung pathology.

Answer 2:

8) **Right apical pneumothorax:** This radiograph is labelled 'Red dot', indicating to the interpreter that the radiographer who took the image believes that the radiograph has pathology present. This ensures that whoever interprets the radiograph is aware that if they cannot find the pathology then they should contact the radiographer or a radiologist. Viewing the lungs bilaterally, it can be seen that the right upper thorax shows no lung markings and the lung edge can be seen at a lower margin, seen as a thin white line, the visceral pleura. This is therefore a pneumothorax as there is free air between the visceral and parietal pleurae. This is not considered to be a tension pneumothorax, as the mediastinum remains central with no shift. Pneumothoraces may be iatrogenic, spontaneous, due to trauma or underlying lung pathology. It is therefore important to continue assessing the radiograph for further lung pathology; however, the lungs in this radiograph are bilaterally clear.

Answer 3:

2) **Congestive cardiac failure:** The hilum is bilaterally prominent and engorged, giving the appearance of 'bats' wings'. There is upper lobe venous prominence from raised pulmonary venous pressure, and definite blunting of the right costophrenic angle, indicating a pleural effusion. Fluid may also be seen in the horizontal fissure. All these signs indicate congestive cardiac failure. Although the heart appears enlarged, the actual size cannot be commented upon accurately, as this is an AP projected radiograph (therefore the heart is magnified).

Answer 4:

10) **Right upper lobe consolidation:** There is an opaque area in the right upper lobe suggestive of consolidation in a lobar configuration, suggestive of a diagnosis of pneumonia. However this should be interpreted carefully in the

context of the clinical picture as malignancies (and other diagnoses) may appear similar. A follow-up chest radiograph to assess for resolution after treatment is essential.

Answer 5:

5) Left lung mass: Likely causes are primary or metastatic malignancies, round pneumonias, lung abscesses and rheumatoid nodules. There may also be additional findings on the radiograph (not shown) depending on the pathology such as a collapsed lung, the presence of pleural effusions, or enlarged lymph nodes if the mass was a bronchial carcinoma for example.

Answer 6:

8) Small bowel obstruction: This plain abdominal radiograph shows dilated loops of bowel in the centre of the film with valvulae conniventes running across the bowel wall. These findings are in keeping with a diagnosis of small bowel obstruction. To remember the potential causes of this think from the inside out, e.g. intraluminal obstructing mass, bowel wall malignancy, adhesions and hernias.

Answer 7:

2) Calculi: This is a KUB (kidneys, ureters, bladder) plain radiograph and is used when renal pathology is suspected. This radiograph shows calcification in both the left renal parenchyma and in the left ureter, strongly suggestive of renal and ureteric calculi.

Answer 8:

4) Large bowel obstruction: This plain abdominal radiograph shows dilated loops of bowel at the periphery of the film with haustra running only partially across the bowel wall. These findings are in keeping with a distal large bowel obstruction. Potential causes include malignancy and diverticular disease.

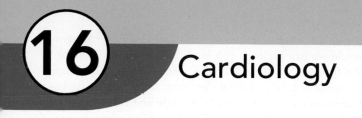

Cardiology

Questions

ELECTROCARDIOGRAM INTERPRETATION: EMQs

For each of the following clinical scenarios, all of which focus on electrocardiogram interpretation, please choose the most important finding shown. Each option may be used once, more than once or not at all.

Diagnostic options

1) Atrial fibrillation
2) Atrial flutter
3) First-degree heart block
4) Second-degree heart block
5) Sinus tachycardia

6) ST segment depression
7) ST segment elevation
8) Third-degree heart block
9) Ventricular fibrillation
10) Ventricular tachycardia

Question 1:

You are the junior doctor on-call over the weekend and a nurse has telephoned asking you to review a 70-year-old man. On arrival, a crash call has already been put out and you are handed the ECG below.

What does the ECG show?

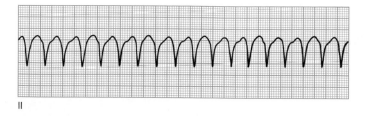

II

Fig. 16.1 Cardiology question 1. Reproduced with permission from Andrew Haughton and David Gray, *Making sense of the ECG.* p. 259. Fig. 17.3.

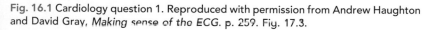

Question 2:

You are a junior doctor working in the accident and emergency department when a 30-year-old woman presents with her husband, complaining of palpitations. She first noticed the palpitations that morning, but became increasingly concerned as by the evening they were still present. Her husband also feels that she has become more irritable recently and commentated on her weight loss. While taking the history you notice she has a slight tremor. An ECG is taken in the department and is shown below.

What does the ECG show?

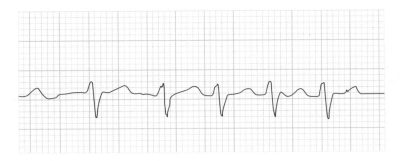

Fig. 16.2 Crdiology question 2.

Question 3:

You are a junior doctor working in the accident and emergency department when a 50-year-old businessman presents complaining of central chest pain. He is known to have hypertension and on examination he is overweight with nicotine stains on the right index and middle fingers. You immediately request an ECG and this is shown in Fig. 16.3.

What does the ECG show?

Question 4:

You are the junior doctor working in the pre-operative assessment clinic and the next patient for you to see is a 60-year-old gentleman. The nurse has already performed an ECG and this is shown in Fig. 16.4.

What does the ECG show?

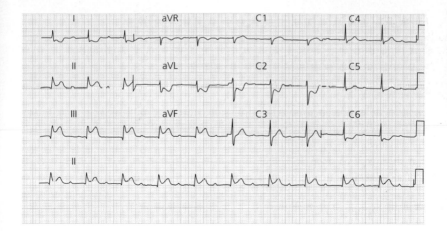

Fig. 16.3 Cardiology question 3.

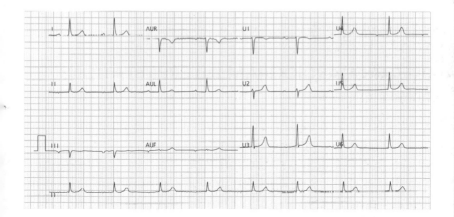

Fig. 16.4 Cardiology question 4.

CHOICE OF INVESTIGATION: SBAs

For the following clinical scenario, please choose the single most appropriate answer from the options given.

Question 5:

You are the junior doctor on the admissions unit and you have been asked to see a 60-year-old woman who presents with shortness of breath. She reports that this has been getting worse over the last few months and that she has noticed that she needs to sleep on three pillows. In addition, she complains of waking up short of breath on occasions. You wish to confirm your clinical suspicion and so request an investigation. Which, from the list below, is the most appropriate?
1) Angiography
2) Echocardiography
3) Nuclear cardiac imaging (Myoview) scan
4) Blood cultures
5) Troponin levels

Answers

ELECTROCARDIOGRAM INTERPRETATION: EMQs

Answer 1:

10) Ventricular tachycardia: Two rhythms which need to be instantly recognisable to any doctor are ventricular tachycardia (VT) and ventricular fibrillation (VF). *Pulseless* VT and VF are cardiac arrest rhythms and require immediate DC cardioversion. VT with a pulse may be found in relatively stable patients and may be treated with drugs, e.g. amiodarone rather than cardioversion in certain situations.

Answer 2:

1) Atrial fibrillation: Note the absence of P waves and the irregularly irregular ventricular rate. This patient, a young female, has symptoms and signs consistent with thyrotoxicosis. Thyrotoxicosis is a known precipitant of atrial fibrillation.

Answer 3:

7) ST segment elevation: This patient has ECG changes diagnostic of an acute inferior ST segment elevation myocardial infarction (STEMI). Note the ST elevation in leads II, III and AVF and reciprocal ST depression in leads I, AVL, V2 and V6. It is important to interpret this ECG correctly so that primary percutaneous coronary intervention can be considered as soon as possible. There is also coexistent first-degree heart block, but that is not the most important finding.

CHOICE OF INVESTIGATION: SBAs

Answer 4:

3) **First-degree heart block:** This is evident from the prolonged PR interval. This can be a normal variant and does not necessarily require intervention. Nonetheless this patient needs to be referred for senior review. There is also bradycardia, but that is not listed as an option.

Answer 5:

2) **Echocardiography:** This patient has symptoms suggestive of heart failure. The NICE guidelines for the diagnosis of heart failure are clear: first perform an ECG and (if available) measure B-type natriuretic peptide (BNP) levels to try to exclude heart failure. If one of these is abnormal then request an echocardiogram. Other investigations (e.g. a plain chest radiograph) should be undertaken to exclude alternative pathologies, but this question asks for the most appropriate investigation to test your clinical suspicion. Blood cultures are incorrect because these are used in the assessment of endocarditis (which is unlikely given the patient's symptoms). Troponin levels would be very useful if this history was in the acute setting, but the problem appears chronic and so an acute myocardial infarction is unlikely (also note the absence of chest pain). Angiography and Myoview scanning are both useful for investigating ischaemic heart disease. Although the heart failure could have an ischaemic aetiology, neither of these would be the first-line diagnostic test in this case.

> **MICRO-refrence**
> National Institute of Clinical Excellence. Chronic heart failure: National Guidelines for diagnosis and management in primary and secondary care. 2010. http://guidance.nice.org.uk/CG108/Guidance/pdf/English (accessed 23/08/2011).

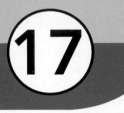

Respiratory

Questions

RESPIRATORY DIAGNOSES: EMQs

For each of the following clinical scenarios, all of which focus on shortness of breath, please choose the most likely diagnosis. Each option may be used once, more than once or not at all.

Diagnostic options

1) Asthma
2) Bronchial carcinoma
3) Congestive cardiac failure
4) Exacerbation of COPD
5) Hypoalbuminaemia

6) Hypothyroidism
7) Pancoast's tumour
8) Pneumonia
9) Pulmonary embolus
10) Tuberculosis

Question 1:

You are the junior doctor on the respiratory ward and have been asked to see a 70-year-old man who was admitted earlier from the community. He is short of breath, which has been worse over the last 2 days, with a cough productive of purulent sputum. From his past medical history you note he has chronic obstructive pulmonary disease (COPD) and gave up smoking 5 years ago. On examination you find him pyrexial with a temperature of 38.8°C. On reviewing his plain chest radiograph you notice a pleural effusion at the left lung base. This is aspirated and appears yellow. The aspirate is reported as having a total protein of 35.3 g/L. What is the most likely cause of this patient's shortness of breath given the findings?

Question 2:

You are the junior doctor on the respiratory ward and have been asked to see a 73-year-old woman who was admitted earlier from the community. She is short of breath, which has been gradually getting worse, particularly when lying flat. On reviewing her plain chest radiograph you notice bilateral pleural effusions. An aspirate is performed and appears straw-coloured. The aspirate is reported as having a total protein of 23 g/L. What is the most likely cause of this patient's shortness of breath given the findings?

Question 3:

You are the junior doctor on the admissions unit when a 30-year-old man, of no fixed address, is admitted to hospital with shortness of breath and a cough productive of blood-stained sputum. On reviewing his plain chest radiograph you notice a right-sided pleural effusion. You send both the sputum and a pleural aspirate to microbiology for analysis. The pleural aspirate is reported as having a total protein of 34.2 g/L. While you wait for the sputum culture, your consultant asks you what the most likely cause of this patient's shortness of breath is given the findings so far.

DIAGNOSTIC INVESTIGATIONS INTERPRETATION: EMQs

For each of the following clinical scenarios, all of which focus on shortness of breath, please choose the most appropriate diagnostic investigation. Each option can be used once, more than once or not at all.

Diagnostic options

1) Bronchoscopy
2) CT pulmonary angiography (CTPA)
3) CT scan
4) D-dimer
5) Peak expiratory flow rate
6) Plain chest radiograph
7) Pleural biopsy
8) Spirometry
9) Sputum culture
10) Ventilation/perfusion (V/Q̇) scan

Question 4:

A 16-year-old female presents to the accident and emergency department acutely short of breath. Her mother informs you that she suffers from asthma and that a relative had brought their dog to the house. You suspect this may be an asthma attack and want to start treatment appropriately. Which investigation would you like to perform first to give you an indication of severity?

Question 5:

You are the junior doctor on-call and have been asked to see a 30-year-old woman who is acutely short of breath. She has mild haemoptysis and a pulse of 125 beats/min. Her medical history reveals that she fractured her leg three weeks ago, which remains in a cast. From the options, what would be the best diagnostic investigation?

LUNG FUNCTION TEST INTERPRETATION: EMQs

For each of the following clinical scenarios, all of which focus on lung function tests, please choose the most likely diagnosis. Each option can be used once, more than once or not at all.

Diagnostic options

1) α_1-Antitrypsin deficiency
2) Asthma
3) Caplan's syndrome
4) Coal worker's pneumoconiosis
5) COPD

6) Farmer's lung
7) Idiopathic pulmonary fibrosis
8) No abnormality
9) Occupational asbestos exposure
10) Pigeon fancier's lung

Question 6:

You are the junior doctor on a respiratory ward and you have been asked to evaluate a 65-year-old man's spirometry results. Of note, he is a former coal miner and complains of arthritis in his hands. The results come back as:

	Results
FEV_1	70% of predicted
FVC	51% of predicted
FEV_1/FVC	86%

What is the most likely cause of these results?

Question 7:

You are the junior doctor on a respiratory ward and you have been asked to evaluate a 65-year-old woman spirometry results. Of note, she is a smoker of 20 cigarettes per day and on examination has a diffuse wheeze. The results come back as:

	Results
FEV_1	41% of predicted
FVC	63% of predicted
FEV_1/FVC	54%

What is the most likely cause of these results?

Question 8:

You are a trainee doctor working in primary care when a 19-year-old male presents complaining of shortness of breath. You ask the nurse to perform spirometry. The results are below and listed as 'results 1'. You administer a β_2-agonist and 30 minutes later you ask for the spirometry to be repeated. The results are below and listed as 'results 2'.

	Results 1	Results 2
FEV$_1$	40% of predicted	86% of predicted
FVC	61% of predicted	91% of predicted
FEV$_1$/FVC	52%	90%

What is the most likely cause of these results?

MANAGEMENT OPTIONS: SBAs

For each of the following clinical scenarios, all of which focus on acutely ill patients, please choose the most appropriate next step from the options below. Select the best single answer, each option may be used once only.

Question 9:

You are the junior doctor on-call and have been asked to see a 60-year-old woman who was admitted under the medical team with worsening shortness of breath and reduced respiratory rate. You find her acutely unwell and notice she is on 40% oxygen via a Venturi mask. A quick glance at the notes reveals that this patient has COPD. Worried, you obtain an arterial blood gas sample for analysis and compare it to the sample taken on admission. The results for both are below.

	ABG on room air on admission	ABG at $FiO_2$40% 1 hour later
pH (NR $= 7.35–7.45$)	7.37	7.29
PaO_2 (NR $= 11–13$ kPa)	6.8 kPa	18.1 kPa
$PaCO_2$ (NR $= 4.7–6.0$ kPa)	5.8 kPa	9.4 kPa
HCO_3 (NR $= 24–30$ mmol/L)	33.0 mmol/L	24.1 mmol/L

NR, normal range.

What would be the most appropriate next-step in her management?
1) Change the Venturi mask and reduce the FiO_2 to 28%
2) Give bicarbonate to raise the pH

3) Stop oxygen therapy
4) Switch oxygen to a flow rate of 2 L/min via nasal cannulae
5) Watch and wait

Question 10:

You are the junior doctor working in the accident and emergency department when a 22-year-old woman presents dehydrated and complaining of generalized abdominal pain. She has a 3-day history of thirst and polyuria. An arterial blood gas sample is obtained and the results are shown below.

pH: 7.27 (normal range 7.35–7.45)
$PaCO_2$: 12.0 kPa (normal range 11–13 kPa)
$PaCO_2$: 2.9 kPa (normal range 4.7–6.0 kPa)
HCO_3^-: 12.3 mmol/L (normal range 24–30 mmol/L)
Base excess: −16.3 mmol/L (normal range −2 to +2 mmol/L)
Anion gap: 27.2 mmol/L (normal range 12–16 mmol/L)

What would you like to do next?
1) Obtain a PEFR reading
2) Obtain a set of blood cultures
3) Request a CT
4) Request a plain chest radiograph
5) Perform a urine dipstick

Answers

RESPIRATORY DIAGNOSES: EMQs

Answer 1:

8) **Pneumonia:** Pneumonia is common in those who have COPD. Also, the aspirate appears yellow, which can suggest an infective cause. Finally, the total protein is above 30 g/L, which classes the fluid as an exudate. The differential diagnosis for an exudative pleural effusion should include malignancy (e.g. bronchial carcinoma, mesothelioma), infection (e.g. pneumonia, tuberculosis) and pulmonary embolus. Although malignancy is also a possibility in this patient, the presence of a pyrexia and yellow aspirate makes this less likely.

Answer 2:

3) Congestive cardiac failure: This elderly woman has a history of orthopnoea. The aspirate appears straw-coloured (which is normal), and finally, the effusions are bilateral with a total protein below 30 g/L. This is therefore classified as a transudate. The differential diagnosis for a transudative pleural effusion should include renal failure, heart failure, liver failure, hypothyroidism and hypoalbuminaemia.

Answer 3:

10) Tuberculosis: Homeless patients are more susceptible to become infected with tuberculosis (TB). The shortness of breath and blood-stained sputum are suggestive of the condition. In addition the pleural aspirate has a total protein above 30 g/L and is therefore classified as an exudate. TB is a cause of an exudative pleural effusion (see answer 1) and would fit with the history. Sputum cultures would help exclude a more common cause of effusion such as pneumonia with a parapneumonic effusion, and can be examined for the presence of acid-fast bacilli and cultured to confirm the diagnosis of TB.

DIAGNOSTIC INVESTIGATIONS INTERPRETATION: EMQs

Answer 4:

5) Peak expiratory flow rate: One of the measures of the severity of an asthma attack is the peak expiratory flow rate (PEFR) (see the BTS guidelines for more information). A PEFR of less than 33% of best or predicated is indicative of a life-threatening attack and a PEFR of between 33% and 50% is indicative of a severe asthma attack. An arterial blood gas sample may also be appropriate in a severe or life-threatening attack to fully assess oxygenation. While spirometry may be useful in assessing reversibility it is not appropriate in the acute setting. A plain chest radiograph may be normal in an acute asthma attack or may show some chest hyperexpansion; however, this will not give you information regarding severity. Nonetheless, it would help rule out an infective cause for the exacerbation. A sputum culture would also be useful to rule out an infective cause, but would not be the most important investigation in the acute setting. A V̇/Q̇ scan would be inappropriate as this is not diagnostic for asthma (which is at the top of the differential diagnosis list in this scenario).

MICRO-refrence

British Thoracic Society. *British Guidelines on the Management of Asthma.* 2008 (revised 2009). http://www.brit-thoracic.org.uk/Portals/0/Clinical%20 Information/Asthma/Guidelines/sign101%20revised%20June%2009.pdf (accessed 26/05/2010).

Self-assessment

Answer 5:

2) CT pulmonary angiography (CTPA) scan: This patient most likely has a pulmonary embolism. Her risk factor, detailed in the history, is the immobilized leg in a cast following a fracture. While ventilation/perfusion scans used to be performed (and in certain circumstances such as pregnancy may still be performed), they have now been superseded by CTPA scans which are more accurate. A plain chest radiograph and/or D-dimer may be suitable in cases where there is a low index of suspicion, but in this case the patient is acutely unwell with a tachycardia and haemoptysis; therefore, a CTPA is more appropriate. Additionally, while a plain chest radiograph can be undertaken to exclude alternative pathologies before subjecting a patient to the higher doses of radiation that occur with CTPA scans, it would not be diagnostic in this case and the question asks for the best diagnostic investigation.

> **MICRO-refrence**
> British Thoracic Society. Standards of Care Committee Pulmonary Embolism Guideline Development Group. BTS guidelines for the management of suspected acute pulmonary embolism. *Thorax* 2008; 58: 470–84.

LUNG FUNCTION TEST INTERPRETATION: EMQs

Answer 6:

3) Caplan's syndrome: The results indicate a restrictive defect, as the FEV_1/FVC ratio exceeds 80% while each individual figure is low. This means that lung capacity is reduced, but that air can be exhaled at a relatively normal rate. This is opposite to what one would expect in patients with airway obstruction. This patient is a former coal miner and also complains of arthritis in his hands (which is probably rheumatoid arthritis (RA)). With this combination this patient is most likely to have Caplan's syndrome (a syndrome which presents with both RA and lung fibrosis). Without the arthritis, then the patient would most likely have coal worker's pneumoconiosis. Conversely, patients with RA may develop pulmonary fibrosis; therefore, in this case the occupation is of paramount importance.

Answer 7:

5) COPD: The results of the spirometry are all low and this is characteristic of an obstructive defect. Given that this woman is 65, smokes, and has a diffuse wheeze the most likely cause for this would be COPD (although asthma is a possibility, it is unlikely to have started now without a prior history). COPD is a combination of emphysema and chronic bronchitis and although generally considered to result in an obstructive defect those in whom emphysema predominates have a restrictive defect. These patients are typically described as the 'pink puffers', as opposed to those in whom chronic bronchitis predominates, which results in an obstructive defect and are hence described as the 'blue bloaters'. There is no evidence in the history to suggest an infective or occupational cause.

Answer 8:

2) **Asthma:** This case demonstrates the typical airway reversibility found in asthma. The patient is young and so COPD is unlikely (only with a family history would one consider α_1-antitrypsin deficiency). Also, the first results show a restrictive pattern whereas the second results are normal. Such reversibility is not seen in COPD. This case stresses the importance of pharmacological management in this condition and the benefit that β_2 agonists can provide.

MANAGEMENT OPTIONS: SBAs

Answer 9:

1) **Change to a Venturi mask and reduce the FiO_2 to 28%:** Hypoxic drive in COPD patients is a highly controversial topic and the advice students receive is often conflicting. Nonetheless it is commonly examined so students should know about it! It is said that COPD patients rely on being in a hypoxic state to drive respiration as they have become used to high levels of CO_2 (in contrast people without COPD rely on rising CO_2). In this clinical presentation it is imperative that an arterial blood gas (ABG) be repeated after 30 minutes following a change in oxygen concentration to assess response to treatment and allow for the correct titration of oxygen. Although hypoxic drive is commonly taught and asked about, always remember that hypoxia kills and so if in doubt give high flow oxygen but repeat the ABG after 30 minutes to ensure a positive response to treatment. Note that although the $PaCO_2$ is higher at 18.1 kPa than before when the patient was on room air, it is low when compared to the high concentration of oxygen being administered (generally the $PaCO_2$ should be 10 lower than the FiO_2 provided).

> **MICRO-refrence**
> O'Driscoll BR, Howard LS, Davison AG. BTS guideline for emergency oxygen use in adult patients. *Thorax* 2008; **63** (Suppl VI): vi1–68.

Self-assessment

Answer 10:

5) **Perform a urine dipstick:** This patient's ABG shows a significant metabolic acidosis with some respiratory compensation. Given the history and the increased anion gap, one must consider diabetic ketoacidosis. The next sensible step in the management of this patient would therefore be to perform a urine dipstick to look for ketones. Although not listed in the options, a Boehringer Mannheim (BM) test and serum blood glucose should also be taken immediately as this will quantify the hyperglycaemia.

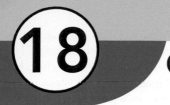

Gastrointestinal

Questions

DIAGNOSTIC INVESTIGATIONS: EMQs

For each of the following clinical scenarios, please choose the most appropriate investigation from the list of options below. Each option can be used once, more than once or not at all.

Diagnostic options

1) Colonoscopy
2) Computed tomography
3) Echocardiography
4) Endoscopic retrograde cholangio-pancreatography (ERCP)
5) Glucose
6) Magnetic resonance imaging
7) Oesophagogastroduodenoscopy (OGD)
8) Plain abdominal radiograph
9) Serum antibodies
10) Serum amylase

Question 1:

You are a trainee doctor working in primary care when a 60-year-old man presents to you complaining of increasing shortness of breath. He notices it particularly when walking up stairs and he comments that it has been getting worse over the last 6 months. He is normally very fit and active with no significant past medical history. You request a full set of simple blood tests, which report the presence of a microcytic hypochromic anaemia (haemoglobin of 8 g/dL). He reports no change in bowel habit. From the above options, what would be the most appropriate next investigation?

Question 2:

You are a junior doctor working in the accident and emergency department when a 55-year-old man presents with epigastric pain radiating into the back along with nausea and vomiting. On questioning he reports that the pain came on while he was eating at a local curry house and consuming alcohol. What would the most appropriate initial investigation?

Question 3:

You are a trainee doctor working in primary care when a 62-year-old man comes to see you complaining of food getting stuck in his throat when he is eating. He has no problems swallowing liquids. He feels he may have lost some weight as his trousers seem looser than normal and his wife also agrees, but neither can quantify an amount. You decide to refer him to the local gastroenterology department but in the meantime you arrange for him to have an investigation. From the list above, what is the most appropriate investigation?

CHOICE OF INVESTIGATION: SBAs

For the following clinical scenarios, please choose the single most appropriate answer from the options given.

Question 4:

You are a trainee doctor working in primary care when a 20-year-old woman presents to you with lethargy and diarrhoea. Her symptoms appear related to her diet and you suspect she may have coeliac disease. You decide to request some blood tests to help support your clinical suspicion. From the options below, which one is the most diagnostic for coeliac disease?

1) B12
2) Folate
3) IgA endomysial antibodies
4) IgA tissue transglutaminase antibodies
5) Iron

Question 5:

You are a trainee doctor working in primary care and have been asked to see a 43-year-old man who has recently joined the GP practice for a new patient assessment. He is new to the area and has not previously engaged with the health services, so there are no previous medical records. On examination you detect splenomegaly, hepatomegaly and signs of chronic liver disease. On direct questioning he denies excessive alcohol consumption. He is not in regular contact with any members of his family, but says that his brother died when he was young from cardiomyopathy and his father died from liver failure. You are naturally concerned, and so organize some investigations. Which of the tests below would be most specific to your suspected diagnosis?

1) Antimitochondrial antibody
2) Caeruloplasmin
3) ESR
4) Ferritin
5) pANCA

Answers

DIAGNOSTIC INVESTIGATIONS: EMQs

Answer 1:

1) Colonoscopy: This patient has iron-deficiency anaemia, suggesting a gastrointestinal malignancy until proven otherwise. The fact that he is reporting no change in bowel habit is not necessarily reassuring. Right-sided bowel malignancies can become very large before they cause a change of bowel habit. Therefore investigation is warranted.

Answer 2:

10) Serum amylase: This patient most likely has pancreatitis as the pain radiates to the back, which is classical for this condition. In addition he has likely had a fat-rich meal and he has admitted to consuming alcohol (one of the most common causes of pancreatitis). Acute pancreatitis results in extremely high concentrations of serum amylase and so this investigation is diagnostic for this condition. Endoscopic retrograde cholangiopancreatography (ERCP) is not appropriate in acute pancreatitis and can actually precipitate an attack. An alternative diagnosis is that of gastritis; however, pain from the stomach less commonly radiates to the back. Were this patient to have gastritis then an oesophagogastroduodenoscopy (OGD) would be the diagnostic investigation. However, the question asks for the initial investigation and a blood test is a lot easier to request than an OGD. A serum amylase is always requested in cases of abdominal pain along with other routine bloods for this very reason (a negative serum amylase result makes acute pancreatitis very unlikely).

Answer 3:

7) Oesophagogastroduodenoscopy: This patient is reporting dysphagia with weight loss. One must be very concerned about the possibility of oesophageal malignancy. An OGD is therefore the most appropriate investigation from the list of options, as it will allow visualization of the upper gastrointestinal tract, and biopsy if required.

CHOICE OF INVESTIGATION: SBAs

Answer 4:

4) IgA tissue transglutaminase antibodies: The NICE guidelines for the assessment of coeliac disease state that when you have a clinical suspicion and the patient has symptoms suggestive of coeliac disease serological testing should be offered. IgA tissue transglutaminase antibodies are the first-choice serological test with IgA endomysial antibodies being tested only if the results of the IgA tissue transglutaminase antibodies are unclear. The other options are all used for investigating malabsorption, but none is specific for coeliac disease.

> **MICRO-refrence**
> National Institute of Clinical Excellence. Coeliac Disease: Recognition and assessment of coeliac disease. 2009. http://www.nice.org.uk/ nicemedia/live/12166/44355/44355.pdf (accessed 30/06/2010).

Answer 5:

4) Ferritin: The most likely diagnosis is hereditary haemochromatosis. This patient's family history is significant, as liver failure and cardiomyopathy are conditions associated with hereditary haemochromatosis. This condition is most commonly found in men and results in iron deposition in multiple organs, indicated by a high serum ferritin level. This is an autosomal recessive condition resulting from a defect in the HFE gene. Genotyping may be performed to confirm the diagnosis.

The alternative answers all suggest other pathologies: antimitochondrial antibodies are diagnostic of primary biliary cirrhosis; pANCA is elevated in primary sclerosing cholangitis; caeruloplasmin is low in Wilson's disease; high ESR is suggestive of autoimmune hepatitis.

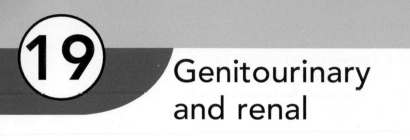

Genitourinary and renal

Questions

DIAGNOSTIC INVESTIGATION INTERPRETATION: SBAs

For the following clinical scenarios, please choose the single most appropriate answer from the options given.

Question 1:

You are a trainee doctor working in primary care when a 20-year-old man presents to you with haematuria and haemoptysis. You suspect that this patient may have Goodpasture's syndrome. You have decided to carry out a diagnostic test. Which from those listed below is this?
1) Anti-nuclear antibody (ANA)
2) Anti-glomerular basement membrane
3) Anti-streptolysin O
4) cANCA (cytoplasmic ANCA)
5) pANCA (perinuclear ANCA)

Question 2:

You are the junior doctor working in the neurology service. A 33-year-old woman presented to the accident and emergency department with a headache, which was subsequently diagnosed as a subarachnoid haemorrhage and managed accordingly. She is recovering well and you take this opportunity to undertake a full history and examination. On abdominal examination you find two ballotable masses. What investigation from the list below is most suitable in the first instance?
1) Biopsy of the mass
2) Computed tomography
3) Magnetic resonance imaging
4) Plain abdominal radiograph
5) Ultrasound scan

Question 3:

You are a trainee doctor working in primary care when a 19-year-old woman presents with dysuria and frequency. From the options below, which investigation would you perform first?

1) Biochemistry sample for urea and electrolytes
2) Full blood count
3) Midstream urine sample for microscopy, culture, and sensitivity
4) Urine dipstick
5) Vaginal swabs

Answers

DIAGNOSTIC INVESTIGATION INTERPRETATION: SBAs

Answer 1:

2) Anti-glomerular basement membrane: This is the diagnostic marker for Goodpasture's syndrome. cANCA is diagnostic for Wegener's granulomatosis and pANCA for polyarteritis nodosa. ANA is suggestive of systemic lupus erythematosus (SLE) and antistreptolysin O of post-streptococcal glomerulonephritis.

Answer 2:

5) Ultrasound scan: This patient's ballotable abdominal masses are likely to be enlarged kidneys and this may represent polycystic kidney disease. There is a known relationship between Berry aneurysms (which can rupture causing subarachnoid haemorrhages) and polycystic kidney disease. The first-choice investigation for an enlarged kidney is an ultrasound scan as it is both non-invasive and confers no radiation risk.

Answer 3:

4) Urine dipstick: This patient's history is suggestive of a urinary tract infection and this question asked for the most appropriate *initial* investigation; hence 'urine dipstick' is correct over 'midstream urine for microscopy, culture, and sensitivity'. Urine dipstick is a simple bedside investigation that can provide valuable clinical information (such as the presence or absence of leucocytes or nitrites). With a positive urine dipstick response, you could empirically start antibiotics to treat the urinary tract infection while awaiting the results of the midstream urine sample (to confirm bacterial growth and antibiotic sensitivity).

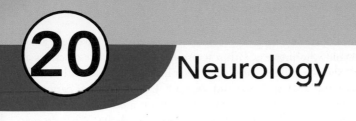

Questions

DIAGNOSTIC INVESTIGATIONS INTERPRETATION: EMQs

For each of the following clinical scenarios, all of which focus on cerebral spinal fluid samples, please choose the most likely findings. Each option may be used once, more than once or not at all.

Diagnostic options

1) Clear cerebral spinal fluid sample, but very low glucose
2) Clear cerebral spinal fluid sample with a high white cell count consisting primarily of lymphocytes
3) Cloudy cerebral spinal fluid sample with a high white cell count consisting primarily of neutrophils

4) Cloudy cerebral spinal fluid sample with a very high glucose
5) High protein concentration
6) Low platelet concentration
7) Low protein concentration
8) Normal
9) Oligoclonal bands
10) Xanthochromia

Question 1:

You are the junior doctor working on the neurology service and a 23-year-old woman patient is admitted complaining of numbness and tingling in her left leg. She says that this is the first time this has happened. On close questioning she also reveals that she was previously admitted with blurred vision that subsequently resolved after a few days. Your seniors request that you send off a cerebral spinal fluid sample a few hours later. What do they suspect might be found?

Question 2:

You are the junior doctor working on the neurology service and have been asked to see a 35-year-old who presents with a severe headache that she describes as 'the worst ever'. She says it feels like she has been hit over the back of her head. Your senior colleagues are concerned and after a CT scan has been performed which was reported as normal, you are asked to obtain a cerebral spinal fluid sample approximately 12 hours after the onset of the headache. What do you suspect might be found?

Question 3:

You are a junior doctor working in the accident and emergency department when an 18-year-old male, first-year university student is brought in unwell, complaining of a headache, pain and stiffness in his neck, and a strong aversion to the light. You are concerned and so organize a head CT (which is reported as normal) which is followed by a lumbar puncture. You suspect that the cause of his disease may be bacterial and look at the results to see if they support your hypothesis. Which option would support your hypothesis?

COMPUTED TOMOGRAPHY INTERPRETATION: EMQs

For each of the following clinical scenarios, please choose the correct diagnosis. Each option may be used once, more than once or not at all.

Diagnostic options

1) Extradural haematoma
2) Foreign body
3) Left parietal infarct
4) Left temporal infarct
5) Metastatic tumour

6) Primary tumour
7) Right parietal infarct
8) Right temporal infarct
9) Subarachnoid haemorrhage
10) Subdural haematoma

Question 4:

You are a junior doctor working in the accident and emergency department and a 73-year-old man presents with recent-onset confusion. When taking the history you find out from his daughter that he has had multiple minor falls over the past few weeks, but that there were no obvious injuries. You decide to request a head CT scan and this is shown in Fig. 20.1.

While awaiting the formal report from the radiologist you review the CT image. What is the diagnosis?

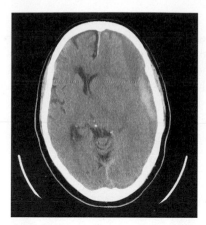

Fig. 20.1 Neurology question 4.

Question 5:

You are a junior doctor working in the accident and emergency department and a 41-year-old woman is brought in following a road traffic incident in which she was a passenger in a car that collided with another. Despite her having a Glasgow Coma Scale score of 15/15 on arrival, you can see from the neurological observation chart that over the last 4 hours this has slowly been declining and is now 11/15. Concerned, you decide to request a head CT scan and this is shown below.

While awaiting the formal report from the radiologist you review the CT image. What is the diagnosis?

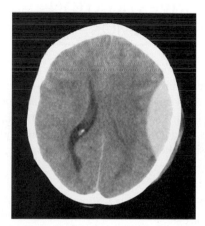

Fig. 20.2 Neurology question 5.

Question 6:

You are the junior doctor working on the care of the elderly ward. A 90-year-old woman has presented with recent-onset left-sided weakness that was first noticed on waking up this morning. A CT scan is requested and is shown below.

While awaiting the formal report from the radiologist you review the CT image. What is the diagnosis?

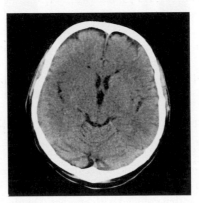

Fig. 20.3 Neurology question 6.

Answers

DIAGNOSTIC INVESTIGATION INTERPRETATION: EMQs

Answer 1:

9) Oligoclonal bands: This patient has new-onset paraesthesia with a history suggestive of at least one episode of optic neuritis. The most likely diagnosis for this patient is multiple sclerosis. Oligoclonal bands of IgG are sometimes found when electrophoresis is undertaken on cerebral spinal fluid samples in patients with multiple sclerosis, although this is not pathognomic.

Answer 2:

10) Xanthochromia: This patient is giving a classical description of a subarachnoid haemorrhage. Xanthochromia results from the breakdown of blood in the cerebral spinal fluid and is best measured after 12 hours from the onset of the headache. It should also be noted that low platelet concentration can never be the correct answer as platelets are not found in the CSF.

Answer 3:

3) Cloudy cerebral spinal fluid sample with a high white cell count consisting primarily of neutrophils: This patient has all the classical features of meningitis (photophobia, neck stiffness and headache), and given his age and occupation it is highly likely that he lives in university halls of residence; this is a significant risk factor for developing bacterial meningitis. On examination of the cerebral spinal fluid from a patient with bacterial meningitis one would expect to find it cloudy with a significantly high protein and low glucose concentration (in comparison with that found in the plasma) with a raised white cell count consisting primarily of neutrophils. In viral meningitis the cerebral spinal fluid sample is typically clear with marginally low glucose and marginally raised protein but with a raised white cell count consisting primarily of lymphocytes.

COMPUTED TOMOGRAPHY INTERPRETATION: EMQs

Answer 4:

10) Subdural haematoma: Subdural haematomas can commonly occur in elderly people following falls that are often considered minor. The CT scan shown is typical of this. It is important to note that subdural haematomas, in contrast to extradural haematomas, can cross suture lines and so form a 'crescent' shape on the CT scan.

Answer 5:

1) Extradural haematoma: Extradural haematomas can occur following blunt trauma. As they develop they can raise the intracranial pressure and subsequently slowly reduce the Glasgow Coma Scale score. The CT scan shown is typical of this. It is important to note that, unlike subdural haematomas, they cannot cross suture lines and form a 'convex' shape on the CT scan.

Answer 6:

8) Right temporal infarct: This woman has had a right middle cerebral artery infarct. The low attenuation in the territory of the right middle cerebral artery is in keeping with an infarct.

Questions

CHOICE OF INVESTIGATION: EMQs

For each of the following clinical scenarios please choose the most appropriate investigation. Each option can be used once, more than once or not at all.

Diagnostic options

1) Alkaline phosphatase
2) Anti-CCP (cyclic citrullinated peptide) antibodies
3) Anticentromere antibodies
4) Anti-double-stranded DNA
5) Calcium pyrophosphate (CPPD) levels
6) Cytoplasmic ANCA (cANCA)
7) C-reactive protein (CRP)
8) Erythrocyte sedimentation rate (ESR)
9) Perinuclear anti-neutrophil cytoplasmic antibodies (pANCA)
10) Uric acid levels

Question 1:

You are a trainee doctor working in primary care when a 41-year-old female patient presents with pain, swelling and stiffness in the small joints of both hands that is worse in the morning and eases during the day. You wish to perform a biochemical test to help predict the progression of this person's disease. Which investigation from the options given would be most appropriate?

Question 2:

You are a trainee doctor working in primary care when a 19-year-old woman presents to you with a rash on her face that appears across the bridge of her nose and below her eyes. Her skin also appears to be particularly sensitive to the light. You suspect you know the diagnosis, but would like to perform an investigation to confirm this. From the list, what would be the most appropriate investigation?

Question 3:

You are a trainee doctor working in primary care when a 52-year-old female presents with cold fingers and toes, deformed digits, swallowing difficulties and telangiectasiae on her face. You suspect you know the diagnosis, but would like to perform an investigation to support this. From the list, what would be the most appropriate investigation?

Question 4:

You are a trainee doctor working in primary care when a 65-year-old woman presents with pain and stiffness in both shoulders, which she has had for some months. She has noticed some weight loss and is generally feeling tired. On examination she has normal muscle power in both shoulders. You suspect you know the diagnosis but would like to perform an investigation to confirm this. From the list, what would be the most appropriate investigation?

FLUID ASPIRATION INTERPRETATION: SBA

For the following clinical scenario, please choose the single most appropriate answer from the options given.

Question 5:

You are a trainee doctor working in primary care when a 70-year-old woman presents with pain in her right wrist and knee. She has a known history of both osteoarthritis and pseudogout. Suspecting pseudogout, a joint fluid aspiration is performed and the sample sent to the laboratory. The result is diagnostic for pseudogout, but what did the laboratory say was seen in the sample?
1) Blood
2) Lymphocytes
3) Negatively birefringent needle-shaped crystals
4) Neutrophils
5) Weakly positively birefringent crystals

CHOICE OF INVESTIGATION: SBA

For the following clinical scenario, please choose the single most appropriate answer from the options given.

Question 6:

Ten days ago you were working as a junior doctor in the accident and emergency department when a 25-year-old man presented with a sore left hand. Earlier that day he had tripped over a roadside kerb and fell with his hands outstretched. Radiographs taken at the time revealed no obvious fracture. You asked to see him again 10 days later. You now wish to perform an investigation. What is this?

1) CT scan of the left hand and wrist
2) Lateral view of the hand
3) Nerve conduction studies
4) Plain radiograph of the left arm
5) Scaphoid series of the left hand

Answers

CHOICE OF INVESTIGATIONS: EMQs

Answer 1:

2) **Anti-CCP (cyclic citrullinated peptide) antibodies:** This patient has symptoms suggestive of rheumatoid arthritis. Anti-CCP antibodies have recently been found to be a more accurate diagnostic test for rheumatoid arthritis than rheumatoid factor (RhF). Research also indicates that the presence of anti-CCP antibodies (especially medium to high concentrations) can give significant prognostic information regarding future joint damage. Although ESR and CRP would also be raised, neither would be diagnostic.

> **MICRO-refrence**
> Quinn MA, Gough AKS, Green MJ, Devlin J, Hensor EMA, Greenstein A, Fraser A, Emery P. Anti-CCP antibodies measured at disease onset help identify seronegative rheumatoid arthritis and predict radiological and functional outcome. *Rheumatology* (oxford) 2006; **45**: 478–80.

Answer 2:

4) **Anti-double-stranded DNA:** This patient has symptoms suggestive of systemic lupus erythematosus (the butterfly rash is classical) and given this, from the list, anti-dsDNA is the most appropriate investigation to perform. Note ESR would usually be elevated in lupus, although CRP is often normal.

Answer 3:

3) **Anticentromere antibodies:** This patient has symptoms suggestive of CREST syndrome (a form of systemic sclerosis) and this is associated with the presence of anticentromere antibodies. CREST stands for calcinosis, Raynaud's syndrome, oesophageal dysmotility, sclerodactyly and telangiectasia.

Answer 4:

8) **Erythrocyte sedimentation rate:** This patient has the classical symptoms of polymyalgia rheumatica. This is characterized by bilateral pain and stiffness in the proximal muscles of the shoulder, but importantly without any evidence of muscle weakness (in contrast with polymyositis). Polymyalgia rheumatica is one of the few conditions that result in very high levels of ESR. Another notable example is giant cell artertitis – a related condition.

FLUID ASPIRATION INTERPRETATION: SBA

Answer 5:

5) **Weakly positively birefringent crystals:** These are diagnostic for pseudogout whilst negatively birefringent needle-shaped crystals are diagnostic of gout. You would not expect the other options in a case of pseudogout.

CHOICE OF INVESTIGATION: SBA

Answer 6:

5) **Scaphoid series of the left hand:** Falling on outstretched hands often results in a scaphoid fracture that may not be seen on radiological examination at the time of injury, therefore it is crucial that this is repeated at 10 days. When investigating for a potential scaphoid fracture it is important to request a 'scaphoid series' as these are a special set of radiographic films that are used to enhance detection of these fractures. The importance of correctly managing a scaphoid fracture is that, due to the blood supply, there is a significant risk of the proximal part of the scaphoid suffering from avascular necrosis.

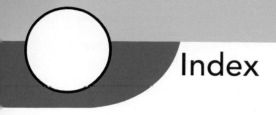

Index

Note: Page numbers with brackets e.g. 211–14(220–3), are to questions with the answer indicated in brackets.

Clinical Investigations